Prepping Parents for Puberty Talks

A Compilation of Over 500 Questions Children Ask
with Child-Friendly Answers

Lori A. Reichel

iUniverse®

PREPPING PARENTS FOR PUBERTY TALKS
A COMPILATION OF OVER 500 QUESTIONS CHILDREN ASK WITH CHILD-FRIENDLY ANSWERS

iUniverse books may be ordered through booksellers or by contacting:

iUniverse
1663 Liberty Drive
Bloomington, IN 47403
www.iuniverse.com
1-800-Authors (1-800-288-4677)

Because of the dynamic nature of the Internet, any web addresses or links contained in this book may have changed since publication and may no longer be valid. The views expressed in this work are solely those of the author and do not necessarily reflect the views of the publisher, and the publisher hereby disclaims any responsibility for them.

Any people depicted in stock imagery provided by Thinkstock are models, and such images are being used for illustrative purposes only.
Certain stock imagery © Thinkstock.

ISBN: 978-1-4917-6450-3 (sc)
ISBN: 978-1-4917-6451-0 (hc)
ISBN: 978-1-4917-6452-7 (e)

Library of Congress Control Number: 2015911969

Print information available on the last page.

iUniverse rev. date: 08/27/2015

For all children who are about to go through,
Are going through,
Or have gone through,
The changes of puberty.

Table of Contents

Acknowledgments

Many people have helped to make this book possible. For the initial edits, I thank Debbie Doucet and Chuck Gunther. Because of the two of you, I was able to reformat initial questions into a reader-friendly manner and order.

Both of my parents, Theresa and Robert Reichel, also read the initial drafts of this book, providing a variety of recommendations. I truly believe that by having my parents read an earlier edition of this book, an opportunity was created to allow us to have conversations that strengthened our relationships. This occurrence serves as an example of how parent-child communication can occur at any age, and I will be forever grateful for this unique occurrence.

I also thank my other family members and friends for their contributions in guiding me with better section titles, the inspiration for completing the final book, and overall general support with "thinking breaks." This includes the following people, listed in alphabetical order to not show favoritism: Aunt Loretta, BRAP, Brian, Bruce, Debby, Debi, Denise, Diane, Dr. Mike, Elyssa, Eric, Farmer Mike, Iris, Jen, Jessica, Joanie Bologna, Joanne, John, Josh, Karen, Kelli, Kevin, Kim, Lily, Maria, Olivia, Renée, Robert, Sandi, Scooter, Stephanie, SusieQ, Uncle Bob, and Uncle John.

In addition, I thank all of the students I have met throughout my teaching years. Each of you reminded me what it was like to be a child again, as well as how important it is to have correct information plus a trusted "puberty expert" in your life.

Introduction: A Letter to Parents

Dear Parent,

Welcome to *Prepping Parents for Puberty Talks: A Compilation of Over 500 Questions Children Ask with Child-Friendly Answers.*

I have written this book to help you, the parent, feel comfortable while talking with your child about puberty. For years, parents have confided in me that talking about puberty with their children causes a variety of uncomfortable feelings. Yet having puberty discussions can create positive opportunities for connecting with your child while helping him/her better understand the journey his/her body and mind is about to take.

Therefore, the goal of this book is simple: to help prepare or "prep" you for puberty discussions with your child. To do this, I have provided over five hundred questions children ask health teachers about puberty. And by reading the questions and provided answers, you will better understand simple and honest ways to engage in conversations with children.

Overall sections within this book include general puberty questions, questions about girls, questions about boys, pregnancy and baby questions, and other relatable questions. I have also included a section for the common questions I have received from parents over the years, as well as suggestions for talking with your child.

By spending the time to engage in honest puberty discussions with your child, both you and your child will not only survive his/her puberty years, yet thrive in your relationship. Remember, you went through puberty.

1

And even if your experience includes sad or anxious memories, think how much better your child's puberty experience will be because you spoke to him/her and shared some of your experiences and lessons. So enjoy the opportunities to communicate and good luck!

I wish you and your child the very best,
Lori A. Reichel

P.S. The term "parent" is used throughout this book to refer to the adult primary caregiver of a child, including the biological parent, other family member, or nonbiological guardian raising a child. Other trusted adults are also referred to and include teachers, counselors, doctors, and other "puberty experts" who can help teach your child.

Questions from Parents

Parents asked the following questions in a variety of settings. They are provided to remind you that parents sometimes experience uncertainty or hesitation in communicating with their child about puberty and other related topics.

When should I talk with my child about puberty?
Parents should speak with their child about puberty at a variety of times. The best time to start is before he/she begins to experience pubertal changes, which may be as early as seven years old for some children. Some parents choose to talk with their child when he/she is in the fourth and fifth grade because, even if their child has not showing physical signs of puberty, some of their child's peers are experiencing changes.

My child has not asked me any questions or made any comments. Should I bring up the topic with her/him?
If your child is approaching the age of puberty, yes, speak with him/her. Some parents think because their child has not said anything to them, they do not need to talk about the topic, yet *this is not true.* Your child may already be curious about what is happening to his/her body or the body of his/her older sibling, cousin, friend, etc..... Starting a conversation when your child is young allows for healthier communication between you and your child. Also, some children are already going through changes, yet their parents are not aware of them.

How do you suggest I approach the topic of puberty with my child?
If your child asks you a question about the topic, you can start having conversations then. However, if he/she has not asked you anything, you

can begin conversations when teachable moments occur. An example of a teachable moment is hearing a message about puberty or sexuality on a television program. Upon seeing/hearing something, a parent can refer to the message and allow his/her child to share thoughts and ask questions. You may also choose to provide a child-friendly book written about puberty to your child and discuss parts of the book with him/her over time.

How many times do I have to talk with my child about this topic?

Parents need to talk about this topic with their child as many times as needed. Some parents think a one-time conversation is enough, but *one conversation is not enough!* Children learn at different rates and, as their bodies continue to change, additional questions arise. Also, because you are raising your child to become independent, future talks can blossom into the emotional and decision-making challenges your child will eventually face, as well as your values and concerns related to sexuality.

I never had anyone talk to me about puberty and I survived it. Why should I talk with my child?

When asked, most young adults admit they wished their parents had spoken with them in an honest and open manner. And, if you think about it, just because you did not have this opportunity does not mean your child should not have it. We are living in a fast-paced world in which the terminology on television, in the movies, and in music has gotten more advanced, and the adult humor more sexual. Young people are hearing and seeing these messages. Therefore, they need adults they can trust (you) to help them better understand these messages, as well as to understand your values.

How can I make sure my child does not do anything sexual?

First, start talking honestly with your child about his/her body when he/she is young. By displaying healthy communication, you are modeling how he/she can approach you with any questions or concerns about this topic (or any other sensitive topic) in the future. And as your child matures and sexual issues or questions arise, share your personal values and hopes with your child. Children admit that the most influential people in their lives are their parents. The bottom line, though, is that you cannot control all of his/her decisions, yet you can positively influence them.

What should I expect when I talk to my child about puberty or sex?

What to expect when talking to your child about this topic depends on many factors, including what he/she has heard from other children and other outside sources, so try to keep an open mind. An analogy I heard years ago explains why an open mind is helpful:

> In regards to the topic of talking to your child about human sexuality, including puberty, there is the good, the bad, and the ugly:
>
> *The good:* You talk with your child about this topic before he/she goes through all of the changes of puberty.
>
> *The bad:* Your child asks you questions you may not have been expecting. Some questions surprise or shock you.
>
> *The ugly:* You answer your child's questions, and your child starts correcting you. Unfortunately, this "ugliness" has happened to some parents because all of us, including your child, are exposed to messages dealing with sexuality. Children have also learned how to find answers to questions through the Internet and their peers.

Although the discussions may be difficult to have at times, your child needs a trusted adult he/she can go to and ask questions. You, his/her parent, are perfect for this.

So talking to my child is "good"? (Sorry for the improper form of English.)

Yes! It is wonderful for you, the parent, to communicate with your child. I have met many parents who thank me for talking with their children during a presentation offered through a school district because they think the presentation will be enough. Yet a one or two-time discussion with a health educator does not allow children to fully comprehend the many aspects of puberty or sexuality. After reading some of the questions asked to teachers, you will understand why I believe this. Your child needs *you* to tell him/her more, especially about *your values*. That is why there is a section in this book titled "Ten Useful Tips for Puberty Talks" to assist you.

Talking to my child may be "bad"?

Not really bad, like in a harmful way, yet "bad" may be your perception of what is going to be or is asked by your child. The reality is if your child feels comfortable with you, different questions will arise. Some may be personal, some may seem advanced for your child, and some you may not be sure how to answer. Also, in my experience, children sometimes ask questions for shock value or to test to see if I really will demonstrate good judgment (this allowed me to get some great practice with my "poker face"). My advice to you is to take your time with the conversation and make sure this is not a one-time talk, but rather the beginning of numerous conversations.

So this can also get "ugly"?

It would be unfair for me not to warn you about this. I have been told many stories from parents about how a conversation suddenly switched to another topic they were not expecting. Remember, children hear things from their peers or older siblings, including on a bus or playground, and see things in the media. Some children look for answers to their questions by searching online. For example, a friend's son, who was eleven years old at the time, did a Google search on his laptop computer for "having babies." Her son was given a list of numerous sites, most dealing with pornography. Imagine his confusion when he was looking for an answer to how babies are made and was shown a pornographic sexual act. Luckily, this mother found out and, with her partner, discussed what their child viewed online. So yes, sometimes unexpected questions, comments, or situations occur, yet parents can correct misinformation and express their values with their children by discussing these occurrences.

What should I do if I am asked a question and do not know how to answer it?

Anytime you do not know an answer to a child's question say, "I don't know, but I will tell you as soon as I find out." Then talk with another adult about the question or read up on the topic from a reliable source, including those noted in the back of this book. When you feel you have an appropriate answer, return to the topic with your child and explain the answer. You may also choose to include your child in your research for the correct answer.

My child has asked certain questions and I am unsure if she is ready for the detailed information. What do I do?

Many parents and educational professionals recommend children first be provided with basic answers to questions. As the conversation continues, monitor your child's body language. If he/she seems satisfied with what is said, you do not need to explain things in more detail. Sometimes children tell a parent that what is said is enough. If your child seems confused or desires more details, ask your child if he/she heard something from another person or what he/she thinks the answer is. By allowing children to share their thoughts, parents can determine how much information to share at that time.

Is this book going to be "over my head" with scientific explanations?

No. The purpose of this book is to supply you with simple child-friendly answers.

Where did these questions come from?

These questions came from my years of experience as a school health teacher speaking with preteens in different settings. Also, some questions are from other health teachers whom I have worked with during this time.

How do children typically ask health teachers these questions?

Usually, children ask questions anonymously on paper, aloud in front of their peers, or after a class lesson.

How have children responded to health teachers' answers?

Due to many health teachers creating a safe environment within the classroom for discussing sensitive topics, children usually respond well realizing the topic is a natural part of life. Many also respond by saying the realities about puberty make more sense to them, and they are not so afraid or worried about what will occur.

What are some questions a school health teacher would not answer?

School health educators are professionals. Usually when the topic is about puberty, the teacher stays on topic. "Off topic" questions are referred to a parent to answer or answered in a small setting when it is appropriate to do so.

Will my school be teaching my child about puberty?

Parents can contact their child's school district to inquire about what puberty lessons are taught because most have board policies about health education. You can also ask the principal and school health teacher at your child's school because they are aware of the sensitive topics being discussed in classes.

Can any teacher teach my child about puberty?

No. School administrators usually make the decision of who will be teaching these lessons to children because it is important for teachers who feel comfortable about this topic to lead the discussions. And, if the school has a health educator, he/she is usually the person to teach this topic. A former peer of mine, who taught sixth graders most of his life, would blush every time I reminded him the topic was being discussed with students in the spring. His comment was usually, "Thank you for doing this… I never could." This statement provides an example of why puberty talks should be presented by adults who feel comfortable with the topic.

Who should answer questions for children?

I tell my preteen audience to ask a trusting person, like a parent, who went through puberty. I call this person a "puberty expert." Talking to a peer who thinks he/she knows the information is not as reliable as an older person who went through the experience.

Is a parent able to teach a child of the opposite sex?

Yes. Just because a parent may not have experienced something does not mean he/she cannot provide information or guidance to a child. If a child wants to talk with someone of the same sex, and that is not you, ask a person you trust to talk with your child.

What commonly occurs during puberty?

Physically: There are many physical changes including growth spurts (height and width), hair growth in new areas, increase in body odor, acne, voice changing, genitals maturing, and overall body shape changes. Also, girls grow breasts, their hips widen, and periods begin (menstruation). For boys, they have more noticeable voice changes, chest hair grows, mature sperm are made, and nocturnal emissions occur.

Emotionally: Many children go through mood changes, in which the statement "my child seems moodier" is commonly stated by parents. This occurrence is not a bad thing —it is a reality. Your child's hormone levels and lives are changing which can create mood swings.

Socially: Children may drift away from spending time with family and start to express their friends as being more important. This change of focus is natural—your child is not going to live with you forever (usually) and a sense of independence occurs during this time of his/her life.

Mentally: Decision-making increases as children age, in which the maturing child needs to understand potential consequences.

Spiritually: Many children also begin to question the values and beliefs taught to them. Doing this allows for value clarification that continues into adulthood.

What feelings do children have about puberty?

Children experience a variety of feelings during puberty. These feelings include happiness, anxiety, fear, frustration, and impatience. Puberty can also cause confusion, so patience, as well as a good sense of humor, is needed by both children and their families

Who can I go to about questions dealing with puberty?

You can talk with your child's doctor, school nurse, counselor, or health teacher. You can also talk with other parents. In addition, there are other resources available for parents, including those listed in the "Resource" section of this book.

Have children ever tried to stump you by asking a question you might not know?

Yes, many children have tried to "stump me." Luckily, I have a great sense of humor and can think on my feet.

What else should I know?

Remember that being a parent requires so many traits: patience, love, patience, strength, patience, and understanding. Did I mention patience? And in this new century, it seems as though your parenting needs to go a little faster. Our children are learning their ABC's earlier, can understand how to download things onto a computer, tablet, or phone better than adults, and are exposed to media messages seeming to mature our children earlier. You have chosen a great job, although it is difficult at times. So give yourself time to process what your child is going through, as well as what you are going through. And remember to get support if you need it because "it takes a village to raise a child."

Is there anything new about preteens and puberty I should be aware of?

Yes. When we start to look at what is going on in our world, we find:

- Some children are beginning to mature physically earlier.
- Children are exposed to an extreme amount of sexual messages in the media, including in/on television programs, movies, music, advertisements, and the Internet.
- Children may be able to ask and talk about sexual topics and behaviors at earlier ages, but they do not fully understand what happens, especially the emotional aspects.

How should I read this book?

Options for reading this book include:

- reading each chapter, one by one;
- skipping ahead to sections more relevant for your child or you;
- skipping around to find the most interesting questions;
- reading the whole book or sections with your child;
- reading the book with another parent or other adult;
- choosing this book as part of a book club; and
- using this book as a resource for parent groups (e.g. Parent-Teacher Organizations).

Note: This book *does not* replace professional help. If you have questions or concerns regarding your child's health, please seek additional support. Your child's doctor, school nurse, health teacher, or school counselor can help guide you to other specialists whose job it is to provide support to parents and children.

Ten Useful Tips for Puberty Talks

1. **Talk at different times with your child.** If you think you only have to talk with your child about this topic one time, compare this number to the thousands, if not millions, of sexual images he/she is exposed to by the time he/she is eighteen years old. One discussion after a presentation at school is not enough. Instead, consider having talks about human sexuality with your child throughout his/her life.

2. **Use a variety of settings to talk with your child.** For example, talks can occur while taking the dog for a walk together or as you are waiting for a movie to start. Many parents also suggest having talks during car rides.

3. **Recognize the differences between your children.** Some children approach their parents with questions while others require their parents to approach them. And some children seem ready to learn information at a younger age while their siblings seem unaware of certain topics or situations. Overall, each child is different and parents need to find the best approach for each child.

4. **Have fun during puberty talks.** By having positive conversations with an occasional giggle, both you and your child will release healthy chemicals that will help to de-stress you. And sometimes a child will be put at ease by hearing about a parent's funny puberty experience and how he/she coped. Just make sure you are not laughing *at* your child or the changes he/she is experiencing during puberty.

5. **Use proper body terminology for reproductive system parts.** Using appropriate medical terms teaches your child positive communication skills while supporting comfort with his/her body. Some people tease and say certain terms, yet using slang terms may support the idea there is something wrong with these body parts.

6. **Be aware that your child might ask personal questions.** If your child asks you a private question, explain to him/her certain information is personal. Doing this demonstrates the value of privacy in which certain personal information is not shared with others.

7. **Think ahead about how you will answer certain personal questions.** Sharing certain personal experiences, like the first time a parent started noticing new body hair growth when he/she was younger, may allow your child to feel more at ease to talk with you. For example, when I tell children about my first experience of shaving my armpits with my father's shaving cream (I smelled like men's cologne all day in school), they are usually put at ease knowing I understand what they are going through. Yet you may need time to figure out what to say when suddenly asked a personal question. If this occurs, tell your child you do not feel comfortable at that moment discussing what he/she asked, while explaining that we all need time to mull certain questions over. Some might disagree with this, yet I would rather have a role model tell a child, "I need to think about your question before I answer you," because this models positive decision-making skills.

8. **Be open-minded and cautious of the "Well, when I was a kid, I never thought about sex" or "I would never have done that,"** etc.... Saying comments like these may stop further communication from your child. Yet you can state, "I would hope you make the best decisions for yourself," and "I feel you are not ready yet." Also, explain your values to your child. By doing this, he/she is more likely to respect them because he/she does not feel threatened to follow them.

9. **Attempt to not put down or tease your child about what they ask.** Teasing can be hurtful, and I know too many children whose parents told other adults about what their child asked in front of him/her.

These children usually do not go back to their parents to ask additional questions.

10. **Use reliable resources.** There are a variety of reliable books and websites available for parents and their children, some of which are listed in the "Resource" section of this book. Many include age-appropriate pictures that can be utilized during puberty conversations. For example, a basic body outline can be printed from a resource for your child to draw pubertal changes he/she expects to occur. Allowing a child to do this is a non-threatening way for your child to share what he/she is already aware of, and allows you to add additional body changes. Another example of using resources is to find age-appropriate diagrams of the male and female reproductive systems to allow your child to visualize body parts and their functions.

Basic "How to" Skills Children Need to Learn

The following skills should be taught to children to allow for an easier transition into adolescence.

For both boys and girls, how to:

- Wash the facial skin, hands, and overall body properly.
- Use deodorant/antiperspirant.
- Shave properly.
- Cope in a healthy manner when experiencing uncomfortable feelings.
- Use assertiveness skills, including how to say "no."
- Communicate effectively with friends, peers, parents, and others.
- Show respect for others, including those different from themselves.
- Follow safety skills, including telling a safe adult about "unsafe" situations or behaviors.

For girls, how to:

- Choose the right sized bra.
- Use menstrual pads or other products during menstruation.
- Dispose of or clean menstrual products properly.

For boys, how to:

- Wear a sports cup or jock strap.
- Wash clothing and sheets after having a wet dream.

Although there are other skills children need to learn, the above skills will help your child cope with basic pubertal changes and new hygienic responsibilities.

General Puberty Questions

The following questions are written in the manner asked by children. Also, the variety of ways children ask the same type of question is shown. Most spelling is correct, yet some errors are left to demonstrate how children sometimes misspell or mispronounce words.

The Basics

What is puberty?
Puberty is the developmental phase of a child's body maturing into an adult's body.

At what age does puberty start? When does all this stuff happen?
Puberty typically begins between the ages of eight and thirteen for girls and the ages nine and fourteen for boys. Yet some children start experiencing changes earlier, as young as seven years old, or as late as sixteen years old.

What is responsible for changing a person's body during puberty?
Chemicals called hormones and genes are responsible for body changes. These hormones include the gonadotropin-releasing hormone (GnRH), the luteinizing hormone (LH), the follicle-stimulating hormone (FSH), estrogen, progesterone, and testosterone. Environmental factors may also trigger pubertal changes.

Why do people have to go through puberty? Why do we need to go through puberty?
Puberty allows everyone's body to become adult size, and if they choose to, have a baby in the future.

Who goes through puberty first- boys or girls?

Girls usually begin pubertal changes earlier than boys.

Why do girls go through puberty before boys? Why do girls grow taller than boys do at our age?

Although both boys and girls have the same chemicals, or hormones, in their bodies creating the changes during puberty, some girls have a release of hormones before boys do.

Why do men go through different changes than women do? Why do men or boys get different things on their body than girls?

Boys go through different changes than girls because they have more of the hormone testosterone creating the "manly" changes, and females have more estrogen and progesterone responsible for the "womanly" changes.

Who goes through more changes, boys or girls? Does everyone have the same "effects" during puberty?

Boys and girls go through many of the same changes, and the different changes, those specific for boys or girls, are almost the same in number.

Does everyone have a growth spurt? Does everyone go through puberty?

Yes, usually everyone goes through puberty. If someone is not showing any physical signs by a certain age, the child's doctor can examine him/her to ensure he/she is a "late bloomer."

Is there anyone who doesn't go through puberty? Can it be possible never to go through puberty?

Although uncommon, some children have growing challenges and are in need of getting help from a doctor.

What is adolescence?

Adolescence is the term used to identify a young person's life during the teenage years.

How long can puberty take? Does it take long to grow up?

How long puberty lasts depends upon the individual. Some children seem to go through the changes quicker than others do, yet puberty takes between two to five years for most youth.

At what age does puberty end?

When puberty ends depends on the person, yet usually by the time a person reaches his/her late teens, most of the pubertal changes and growth have occurred. An individual's body, though, will always be making new cells for other growth and change.

When will I grow taller?

A child begins to grow taller when certain hormones are released and his/her body receives messages from his/her brain telling the body to grow.

How can I grow taller faster?

A child may want to grow taller at an earlier age, yet has to be patient with his/her body because it will grow at the speed it is meant to grow.

I saw a man who was two feet tall. What happened?

A man or woman whose adult height is two feet was born with dwarfism, in which his/her body parts are proportional to his/her height. People with this medical occurrence live typical lives, going to school, getting jobs, and having friends and families.

How can you control body changes (puberty)?

Pubertal changes are part of the natural process of growing older. Young people need to remember everyone is different and, just like a person is unable to control the speed of popping popcorn kernels, a person cannot control the changes or speed of puberty. Yet children can choose healthy behaviors to cope.

I heard steroids help with muscle growth for some children. Is it okay to take these?

A person should only take steroids when it is medically necessary and under a doctor's care because taking steroids when unnecessary and unsupervised can cause damage to a person's body.

Do cats and dogs go through puberty?

Cats and dogs go through their own types of growth cycles to become adult cats and dogs. If you think about it, when comparing the size of a kitten to a fully-grown cat, the cat is noticeably larger. Yet these pets do not have the same challenges of puberty. For example, our pets do not experience pimples.

What changes when people go through puberty?

The most noticeable pubertal changes are the physical ones, making a child's body more adult-like. These changes include his/her body getting larger, body odor increasing, sexual organs maturing, hair growing in different or new places, his/her voice changing, and acne developing. Other changes also occur which are not as obvious. For example, a person may notice changes when dealing with emotions and making decisions, within relationships, and with his/her values. These changes may seem like a lot, yet they happen over time.

Will shorter kids ever be tall?

Many children, even shorter ones, grow taller, yet this takes time. What determines a person's height is his/her body and genetics.

Does how tall you get only depend on how tall your parents are?

A boy or girl may grow to his/her parent's height, yet nothing is definite. How a body grows is unique to the person and he/she may be shorter, as tall, or taller than his/her parents.

My doctor said I would grow to be 5'4". Will that happen?

Maybe. Sometimes doctors predict a child's final height, yet what he/she says is not definite. So a person can take the prediction as a possibility, yet this does not mean it will happen.

Can you have puberty when you're a baby?

No, a person does not go through puberty when he/she is a baby. After birth, the baby goes through the developmental stage of infancy, which is another time of change. *(If a child states he/she saw a baby on television or on the Internet who went through puberty, please discuss this unusual situation with your child. The amount of information children are exposed to can confuse them and we, as adults, need to help them better understand what they have seen or heard.)*

Will you get skinny if you are chubby as a kid?

A person's body size partially depends upon his/her genetics, in which some people are genetically larger than others. Yet what is most important is not necessarily size, but keeping your body healthy by practicing positive habits like exercising and eating well.

I feel chubby. Is this normal?

Many children going through puberty feel "chubby" because of the release of hormones making changes in their bodies. If a boy or girl is concerned about getting heavier, he/she can practice healthy habits and talk with a parent or other trusted adult.

What if I really am fat?

If a boy or girl is concerned about being too heavy, he/she can ask a parent to take him/her to the doctor for a check-up. If a doctor discovers he/she is above a recommended weight, the boy or girl may be guided to follow healthy habits including regular exercise and healthy eating. Remember, though, weight is only one measurement of a person's body and there are other ways to determine the wellness of a person.

Why do doctors check you?

It is recommended for people of all ages, children and adults, to get yearly checkups by a doctor. Just like a car gets checked periodically to help it run efficiently, a person should get his/her body checked to ensure everything is running well. During a checkup, the doctor will listen to the person's heart beating, check his/her weight, height, and blood pressure, and look into his/her ears and eyes. Doctors may also check his/her back to ensure proper alignment of the spine or perform additional tests.

Can I ask my doctor questions during a checkup?

Yes, a person has the right to ask his/her doctor questions while getting a checkup. Just like it is important to have good communication with family members and friends, it is also important to communicate with any doctor a person visits.

Do your eyes grow bigger during puberty?

All parts of a person's body grow proportionately including the eyes. By the time a child finishes going through the body changes during puberty, his/her eyes will be the size they will basically remain for the adult years.

Will I sleep more as a teenager?

Many parents notice their children sleeping later and longer during their adolescent years. This behavior is typical and usually okay because a young person's sleep cycle changes during puberty, and it is important to ensure he/she is getting enough sleep. Changing sleeping habits does not mean, though, that a teenager should sleep all day and night.

My teenage sister hardly gets any sleep. She says that she has too much schoolwork and activities to do. Is that okay?

Unfortunately, some teenagers do not listen to their bodies and get less sleep. Getting less sleep weakens the immune system and affects the brain's job, including being able to pay attention in class. As much as some teenagers think they cannot get a full night's sleep, they need to each night.

What happens after puberty – does anything thing else happen?

Once a person's body has reached his/her adult size, his/her overall body size with basic bone structure will be completed. His/her body, though, continues to create new cells for daily growth of body parts, like hair and nails, or replenishing of cells. Other types of growth also continue including social, mental, emotional, and spiritual changes.

What's that Stink? (Body Odor)

What causes body odor? Do you get body odor from sweating?

Body odor is the smell created by the combination of sweat and typical bacteria. During puberty, the sweat glands become more active, making a person sweat more.

Where are the most common places with body odor?

Any part of the body can get smelly due to sweat combining with bacteria and a person not washing properly. Yet the typical smelly areas are the armpits and feet.

Why are my armpits beginning to smell a lot?

During puberty, the armpit glands and skin become "activated," making the area sweat more. When the sweat combines with bacteria, a smell is formed.

Can people smell my armpit smells?

If your armpit areas have an unpleasant scent, people usually can detect it if they stand or pass by you. Just ask any fifth grade teacher what his/her classroom smells like after recreation time and he/she will probably say there is a sweaty, unpleasant smell in the air due to some students sweating.

How do I stop my armpits from smelling bad?

To prevent smelling bad, a person can wash his/her armpits regularly with soap and warm water. Some children take showers in the morning and then again later in the day, or wash their armpits again later with washcloths. Others, if they are allowed to, wear deodorant/antiperspirant.

What is the difference between deodorant and antiperspirant? How does deodorant help the odor under your armpits? What does deodorant do to stop the sweat?

Deodorant is a product used to cover up underarm odor with a particular scent. In other words, it will "de-odor" stinky scents with a pleasant smell. When buying a deodorant, the person should smell it to ensure he/she likes the scent. Antiperspirant contains a chemical to prevent a person from sweating and does not usually have a scent unless it is combined with a deodorant.

Where are deodorants and antiperspirants applied?

Deodorants and antiperspirants are rubbed into the armpit areas.

Should I test the deodorant before wearing it?

Yes, a person should test any new product on his/her body by first rubbing some of the product onto his/her inner forearm area. He/she should then wait forty-eight hours (two days) to see if his/her skin has a reaction to the product.

When do you use deodorant and antiperspirant?

Underarm products are typically applied after cleaning the armpit areas and before getting dressed for school or work.

At what age should you start wearing deodorant or antiperspirant?

There is no exact age to start wearing deodorant/antiperspirant. If a person begins to sweat or smell more, he/she can begin wearing deodorant/antiperspirant, yet should first talk with a parent for permission.

Do I have to use deodorant /antiperspirant?

No. If a person does not use deodorant/antiperspirant, he/she needs to shower/bathe regularly, especially when going through puberty. Also, he/she should make sure to wear clean clothing and to clean the armpit areas with soap and water after exercising.

I heard that antiperspirant causes cancer. Is that true?

There have been some statements like this on the Internet and news, yet it is debatable. To figure out if he/she should use antiperspirant, a young person should talk with a parent or other trusted adult.

Do people get embarrassed having deodorant and other private stuff in their lockers?

At first a person may feel embarrassed, but when he/she realizes many other people keep personal hygiene products like this in their lockers or backpacks, the embarrassment goes away.

How often are you supposed to change your underwear?

A person should change his/her underwear every day. Underwear may also need to be changed more often if the person is sick (for example, has diarrhea) or just exercised and is sweaty.

Why is it important to keep clean?

Keeping clean helps to lower the amount of germs, including bacteria, on a person's body. And lowering the amount of germs and dirt lessens the chances of smelling yucky, getting sick, and getting pimples.

Hairy Situations for both Boys and Girls (Hair Growth)

Where does hair grow on the body during puberty? Where will I grow hair?

Hair grows in a variety of places for boys and girls, including the armpit and private areas. For the hair on the arms and legs, the lighter hair children have may become darker and thicker. In addition, many boys grow hair on their face, chest, stomach, and back.

How old are you when you grow other hair?

Hair growth can occur as early as eight for some girls, yet it usually occurs around age eleven or twelve for both boys and girls.

How much hair will I grow?

How much hair growth occurs depends upon the individual. A child can ask his/her family members, though, about their experiences because he/she may experience the same growth.

Is hair growth in certain spots, like the private area, natural?

Yes, new hair growth is part of the natural process of going through puberty.

Why do you get hair in your armpits?

Armpit hair helps to wick moisture away so the armpit skin areas are kept dry, lowering the chances of smelly bacterial growth.

Why do you grow hair in other places of the body?

Hair grows in other locations on the body because of the hormones being released during puberty.

Why do you get pubic hair? Why do you get hair by your privates?

Adrenarche, the growth of pubic hair, has been a part of being human for thousands of years and there are many existing theories for why this happens. One theory is cave people needed their private areas to be kept warm during cold weather (remember, underwear was not worn during cave people times). Another theory is pubic hair helps to keep germs away from the private area's openings, including the urethra, vaginal opening, and rectum. And another suggestion is pubic hair has certain scents called pheromones to help people feel attracted to someone.

Why do men grow more hair on their body than women?

Males have more of the hormone testosterone than females which increases hair growth on some areas of their bodies.

When should you start shaving?

When a person should begin to shave depends upon his/her family and his/her maturity level. Therefore, it is recommended a child speak with a parent, older sibling, or another trusted puberty expert upon discovering new or more hair growth. And, if it is decided the hair can be removed, a person who has shaving experience should teach him/her how to shave.

Does everyone shave new hair growth?

No. Some families, including those of particular cultures, do not agree on removing hair from certain body areas while other families do.

What is alopecia?

Alopecia is a medical condition creating hair loss. This hair loss can occur anywhere on the body, yet it most often occurs on a person's head. When this occurs, there are special doctors a person can visit for help.

One Zit, Two Zits, Three Zits, Pop? No! (Acne)

What is acne?

Acne is a skin condition in which bumps form on the outer layer of the skin. It is caused when the pores of a person's skin are clogged by dead skin cells, bacteria, and sebum.

What are pimples?

Pimples are bumps formed on the top of the skin and are a slang term for acne. Other slang terms for acne are zits, whiteheads, blackheads, and skin cysts.

What is sebum?

Sebum is the natural oil made by the sebaceous glands in the skin to lubricate the hair and skin.

Where can you get pimples? Do you get pimples on your face when you go through puberty? Do zits or pimples grow in certain other places besides the face?

Pimples can develop on any skin including the face, neck, shoulders, arms, upper and lower back, and chest. Many children get facial pimples at some point during puberty.

Why do some children or teens get pimples during puberty?

Pimples occur during puberty because of hormonal changes. Many children begin noticing their face feeling oily during the day, which means the skin's sebaceous glands are lubricating the hair and skin of the face, giving a slippery or oily feel. This lubrication attracts more dirt, clogging the skin's pores, and causes pimples.

Do you get pimples from eating sweets?

Eating unhealthy food has not been proven to cause pimples, yet some people notice their acne being worse when eating certain unhealthy foods. Doctors recommend children drink enough water and eat healthy foods because these habits allow for a healthier complexion, including a healthy glow to the skin.

How do you prevent pimples?

A person can do the following to prevent pimples:

- Wash his/her face two or three times a day with warm water and soap. A washcloth can be used gently, yet rubbing the facial skin too hard can cause irritation and redness.

- Be cautious of touching his/her face. Hands have germs and dirt on them so touching the face deposits these germs and dirt onto the skin, increasing the chances of clogging pores. For example, when someone seems to be getting bored, he/she may rest his/her head on his/her hand. This person may then notice pimples, or more pimples, in that area because of this touching.

- Clean the skin area under bangs regularly, including after participating in an activity (for example, exercising). Bangs covering the forehead can further increase the chances of dirt and sweat going into the forehead pores, therefore creating pimples in that area.

- Clean hats, including baseball caps, regularly.

Does stress cause pimples?

The relationship between stress and pimples has many factors to consider. For example, does stress cause pimples or do people's habits when under stress cause pimples? What we do know is a higher level of stress increases the release of cortisol and the production of the natural skin oil, sebum, which may increase the growth of pimples. Also, high levels of stress can negatively affect the immune system, slowing down healing, including the healing of pimples. Yet people may also choose unhealthy habits when under stress, like getting less sleep and eating unhealthy foods, which may also influence the occurrence and severity of pimples.

How do you get rid of acne? How do you stop pimples?

The first step for getting rid of acne is to keep the facial skin clean with regular washing. If acne seems to be a significant concern, a parent can purchase an over-the-counter product containing salicylic acid or benzoyl peroxide for his/her child. These products may help to prevent or clear up acne in which a person needs to follow the directions carefully, including testing the product on his/her forearm beforehand to ensure he/she is not allergic to or irritated by the product. There are also natural organic products and treatments available.

My brother went to a doctor for his acne. Why?

Some people go to special doctors who help with skin conditions. These doctors are called dermatologists and offer other suggestions for getting rid of acne.

My mom tells me to put toothpaste on acne. Is that okay?

Some types of toothpaste contain certain ingredients that dry out the skin. Dermatologists do not usually recommend this, though, because toothpaste can cause rashes on the skin.

Should I pop a pimple/zit?

No, popping a pimple is not recommended because doing this can allow other bacteria or dirt to go into the pore and, possibly, cause scarring of the skin tissue.

From Happy to Sad in Three Seconds (Feelings about and during Puberty)

This topic (puberty) scares me.

The topic of puberty may seem scary, yet once a person experiences puberty, he/she will understand these changes are not bad yet are a part of growing up and becoming a teenager and an adult.

Why does this topic make me feel so weird?

Talking about this topic may make you feel weird because:

    a. you may have never spoken to someone about the topic before, so talking about it is new;

    b. puberty deals with private parts and some people feel uncomfortable talking about these parts at first;

    c. people sometimes tease about this topic; or

    d. any/all of the above.

I am nervous about puberty, and it's hard to talk with my mom. What do I do?

Some people are nervous to talk about puberty, yet talking with someone you trust and respect, like a parent, helps to get rid of or lessen the nervousness. One way to approach a parent is to start the conversation by saying, "Mom/Dad, I want to talk with you, yet I feel nervous." Also, before talking to a parent, the person can write down his/her questions and comments and then refer to these when talking with a parent.

I want to talk with someone about puberty, but I don't feel comfortable talking to my parent. What should I do?

Although you may not feel comfortable at first, a parent can be a positive person to talk with about puberty. Yet if you are unable to talk with a parent, you can find another trusted adult or puberty expert.

What is a puberty expert?

A puberty expert is a trusted person who has experienced puberty and can share information and his/her experiences with a younger person. An example of a puberty expert is an older sibling or cousin, a teacher, a coach, or a counselor.

Why do we get mood swings?

Mood swings happen because chemicals, known as hormones, change in a young person's body. Trying to do too much or not getting enough sleep can increase this occurrence.

Do mood swings differ for boys and girls?

Both boys and girls experience mood swings because both experience hormonal changes during puberty. Upon reaching a certain age, boys get mood swings because their testosterone level goes up, then down, during the day. For girls having regular menstrual cycles, certain hormones will go up for a few weeks and then go down right before they start menstruating.

Do adults get mood swings?

Yes, adults also get mood swings, although some adults do not admit to getting them.

How do I deal with mood swings?

For dealing with mood swings, the first step is to recognize you are experiencing a mood swing or a feeling you do not enjoy. Upon realizing this, you then need to figure out a strategy for how to feel better. Some strategies include writing in a journal, reading, playing music or an instrument, and being physically active.

I'm scared. I've been feeling awkward, and I don't know what to do (and I don't get mood swings). What should I do?

It is common for children to feel awkward or weird at this time of life. Hormones are being released in the body during puberty, which can make a person feel "not himself/herself." When feeling this way, he/she needs to do something healthy to cope. Healthy coping activities include going for a run or bike ride, listening to his/her favorite music, talking to a family member or friend, playing with a pet, or talking with a person he/she trusts.

I am depressed all of the time. Is that normal?

If a young person is depressed or sad and it lasts for more than a few days, the young person needs to talk with a trusted adult, including a parent. Feelings of depression occur in all people, yet usually last for only a short period of time for typical puberty moodiness.

Other Curious Questions

Why are we learning about puberty?

Children learn about puberty to understand the changes they will be going through during their preteen years. Being told about these changes ahead of time helps to reassure a young person that what he/she is experiencing is typical for children during their pre-teen and teen years.

Whose voice changes, boys or girls?

Both boys and girls experience voice changes because both have larynxes that grow. Yet this occurrence is more noticeable with boys because they have higher levels of testosterone creating larger larynxes. For girls, the changes are so small that there may be no noticeable differences in the girls' voices.

At what age does your voice change?

Like other changes, when a person's voice changes depends upon the individual. A typical age to notice voice changes in boys is between thirteen and sixteen.

Is it true everyone came from two cells?

Both boys and girls are made up of cells originally made from two main cells called a sperm (from a male) and an egg (from a female). When a sperm combines with an egg, it is called fertilization. These two cells then continuously divide to make millions of cells.

Why don't boys and girls have the same parts, like vaginas?

Boys and girls do not have the same body parts because of a chromosome found in the father's sperm. This chromosome is either an "XX" or an "XY." Girls are created from the "XX" chromosome and boys are created from the "XY" chromosome.

Is it possible to get boy and girl parts? Is it possible for a girl or boy to have the other gender's body part?

Although this is uncommon, a baby may be born with parts of both male and female genitals. At one point in the person's life, a procedure may be done to have only specific parts remain.

How do people react to their pubertal changes?

Some people feel comfortable about pubertal changes because they understand it is a part of growing up. Some feel nervous or afraid because they are experiencing something new in their bodies. Some are excited because they know they are getting older. And some have a combination of feelings. Whatever a person is feeling is okay, though, because feelings are a part of life and people need to allow themselves time to adjust to these changes, as well as learn how to cope in healthy ways.

Why do most people change their behavior when going through adolescence? Why does my older brother act differently than he used to?

Behavior change is a part of growth and includes becoming more emotionally mature. Examples of this change are adolescents wanting and having increased responsibilities and acting more adult-like. Adolescents can also question ideas or people more which helps them to figure out who they are and want to become.

Why do people who go through adolescence start getting more independent?

Adolescents become more independent than they used to be because they are getting older and making more decisions for themselves. This independence is a part of maturing and learning to take care of oneself.

Are there any "samples" of things that children should get, like deodorants?

Sometimes schools or doctors' offices have free samples or informational booklets for preteens, yet this depends where the person lives and goes to school.

Why do some boys and girls fall in love overnight?

Some boys and girls feel they fall in love with another person during their puberty years because they begin to discover what type of people they are attracted to. Phrases used to describe this attraction include "having a crush" and experiencing "puppy love." Love, though, does not usually happen overnight for two people. "Crushes" can happen quickly, and anything that starts quickly can also end quickly. *(Upon being asked this question, please talk with your child about your values regarding relationships. Children see many images and myths about love in movies and on television, so talking with a parent regarding this topic is important.)*

What happens if people make fun of you during puberty?

Although some people may think it is funny to make comments about others, if what people are saying or doing hurts a person's feelings, it is considered bullying or harassing behavior. The person being "made fun of" needs to tell a trusted adult both at home and at school. At school, teachers and other school personnel should stop this unhealthy behavior and support the person being "made fun of."

When girls and boys go for the "talk" at school, are they going to talk about sex?

The "talks" occurring during the elementary school-age years are usually about puberty and what to expect during this time of life. The topic of sex may be raised, but how much will be discussed depends on who is there, the readiness and maturity level of the boys and girls, and school policy.

Do girls have to learn about boys? Do boys have to learn about girls?

Learning about the opposite sex and their pubertal changes depends upon who is talking with you about puberty. Yet because both boys and girls live on the same planet, learning about both helps you to better understand each other and get along better.

Prepping Reminders

Both boys and girls experience the following changes during their pubescent years:

- beginning or increasing body odor;
- new hair growth;
- acne; and
- moodiness.

Regarding these changes, if your child is naturally curious and asks you questions, it is best to answer them when they arise. For children who seem unaware or disinterested in puberty, it is recommended for you to approach your child before he/she experiences changes. Doing this models positive communication skills.

Questions about Girls

The following questions are written in the manner of how children ask about situations pertaining to girls. Some questions may seem to be repeated, yet the author desires parents to understand the variety of ways children can ask the same question. Most spelling is correct, yet some errors are left to demonstrate how children sometimes misspell or mispronounce words.

Growth Spurts

When do girls start to go through puberty?
Most girls begin puberty between the ages of eight and thirteen.

How do girls know when they have reached puberty?
Girls know they are going through puberty when they notice a change in body shape, including breast development and wider hips, a growth spurt in height, a smelly body odor, hair growth in new places, and/or acne. They also begin their mentstrual cycle.

Why do women have wider hips? Why do girls' hips widen?
Girls' hips widen to create a woman's body, so as a girl begins to grow taller, her body becomes proportionately wider. And, if she becomes pregnant, a woman's wider hips allow more space to carry the baby inside her uterus.

Do our hips widen or do our hipbones widen?
Both of these occur. Hips get wider as girls grow taller and the hip bones grow to help support the body.

I heard that a girl's body might get curvy as she goes through puberty. As curvy, does that mean fat?

As a girl goes through puberty, her figure gets curvier due to the widening of her hips and development of her breasts. Having curves does not mean a girl is fat; having curves means she has a curvy body structure.

Does the vagina get bigger?

Yes, as a child grows, all parts of his/her body get bigger to make body parts proportional. For example, just like a girl's foot grows as she gets older, her vaginal area grows too.

Should I go on a diet to make sure that I do not get fat during puberty?

Girls should be careful of diets because some diets include unhealthy habits that hurt the body, changing how it utilizes food. Instead, girls should try to eat as healthy as possible, including eating fruits, vegetables, and whole grains, and exercising regularly. By creating healthier habits when younger, girls will most likely continue them as they age.

I feel chubby and heard there is a quick way to lose weight. Should I do this?

No. Any product or program advertised as a quick way to lose weight is usually unhealthy and will not keep weight off. It is smarter for people to eat healthier foods, exercise, and learn to appreciate their body shape.

Some girls are skinnier than I am. How can I get that way?

Girls have different body shapes in which some are naturally slimmer and others are naturally curvier. Instead of comparing body shapes, it is more important for girls to take care of their bodies by following healthy habits and accepting their body shape. Each girl needs to learn to love herself and her body.

Budding into Breasts

What are breasts?

Breasts are part of a female's body located in the chest area. They consist of fat, muscles, and milk glands.

What are the nicknames for breasts? Is "tits" a nickname for breasts?

Slang terms, or nicknames, for breasts include "boobs," "boobies," "titties," "tits," "jugs," and "hooters." The term breast is the proper name and is recommended to be used to show respect to others.

Why are there nicknames for breasts?

Nicknames exist because some people were never taught proper terminology and medically accurate information about certain body parts. Also, some people think it is funny to say certain nicknames for body parts.

Why do girls have breasts?

Females have breasts because of different hormones in their bodies. And, if a female chooses to have a baby, the baby can receive breast milk from her breasts.

Can my breasts make milk now? Why do your breasts have milk now?

Young girls do not have milk in their breasts. Only after giving birth to a baby is breast milk made by a female's breasts.

Are bigger breasts better for babies?

No, breast size is unimportant for the creation of breast milk.

Are bigger breasts better?

No, bigger breasts are not better. No breast size is "better" than another breast size.

Do boobs just get big one day?

No, breasts develop over time. First the nipple areas grow outward, forming two larger areas called "buds." As time passes, fatty tissue surrounds the "budding" areas to form breasts.

Why do I have small boobs one day and overnight they are larger?

Although it may seem as though breasts grow overnight, they do not. Breast development takes time. Yet girls may notice certain shirts becoming tighter in the chest area over a short period of time as they continue going through puberty.

My friends have different sizes of breasts. Some have larger and others have smaller breasts. Is that normal?

Yes, it is normal for girls to have different breast sizes. Just as it is normal for girls to have different heights and weights, specific body parts on girls, like breasts, also differ in size.

At what age do most girls develop their breasts?

Breast development depends upon a girl's stage of puberty. You may notice some fourth grade girls getting a little larger in the nipple area of their chest; these girls are early "bloomers" developing breasts before their peers. Other girls will develop breasts later in the fifth, sixth, and older grades.

Do growing breasts earlier make you have bigger breasts?

No, when a girl's breasts begin to develop does not determine their final size.

I was told that if I do certain exercises my breasts would grow bigger. Is this true?

No. A girl can do upper body exercises to strengthen her chest muscles and improve her posture, but no exercise will increase her breast size.

I want big boobs... What can I do?

Girls cannot make their breasts grow bigger than their natural size. And girls who want bigger breasts need to ask themselves why they want them. Is it because they think bigger breasts will make them better? Is it because they think they will get more attention from others? The reality is that having larger breasts does not mean a girl will have more friends or is more of a female. Instead, accepting her body and liking who she is will help others to like and respect her.

Is it normal for my breasts to hurt, like to feel pressure on them and for them to be hard? Does that mean they are growing?

Many girls report feeling pressure or soreness in their chest area as their breasts begin to develop. And, at the beginning stages of breast development, the nipple area forms a "bud" which will feel hard.

I am afraid that something is wrong with my breasts. My breasts hurt me. What should I do?

If a girl is concerned about any part of her body, including her breasts, she should talk with a parent or other trusted adult. She may even ask to have a doctor check her breast development to put her mind at ease.

Why are my boobs sore sometimes before my period?

Some girls have sore breasts a few days before getting their monthly period because of changes in hormone levels. As soon as the period begins, the soreness usually stops. If the soreness does not go away after a few days, a girl should talk with a parent or other trusted adult who may then take her to a doctor for a checkup.

Can smaller boobs be sore too?

Yes, smaller breasts can get sore too.

What should I do about sore boobs?

To ease the pain of sore breasts, girls should wear properly fitted and supportive bras. Some girls choose to wear sports bras when their breasts are sore because these bras limit the movement of the breasts.

Can I exercise if my breasts are sore?

Yes, girls can still exercise even when their breasts are sore, in which this soreness may go away after a few minutes of exercise.

How can I still exercise if my boobs are sore?

Girls can wear supportive bras while exercising to ease soreness. Some girls choose to participate in low-impact exercises, like yoga, to limit how much their breasts will "bounce" and, therefore, limit additional soreness. Other girls, like those who do aerobic exercises, wear sports bras. And girls with larger breasts may choose to wear two sports bras, one on top of the other.

When should you wear a bra?

A girl should wear a bra when she notices her nipples growing larger and fatty tissue starting to appear in her breast area.

How do you know when you need a bigger sized bra?

A good fitting bra should lay smoothly on a girl's body, so if her breasts are being pushed out of her bra, hanging over the sides, a girl needs a larger sized bra.

How do you find the right sized bra?

A girl can find a good fitting bra by properly measuring for one. Directions on how to do this are found on-line, and a parent or other trusted adult can help. Another option is for the girl go get measured for a bra by a woman trained to do so. Many women who work in bra stores or the bra section of department stores are trained to do this.

Won't it be weird to get my chest measured by a stranger?

A girl may feel weird at first, but the woman measuring her chest area should be trained in this skill. To help her feel more at ease, a girl can ask a parent or a friend to stay with her as she is being measured.

What is a typical boob size?

Breasts come in all different shapes and sizes, so a typical "boob" or breast size does not exist.

What are double "D's?

Double "D's" is a size for larger breasts. There are bras made for this size of breasts, as well as for other sizes.

What size bra will I need when I get my period?

There is no definite bra size a girl needs to wear when she gets her period. Instead, she needs to wear a bra that fits her best.

I saw a model wearing a bra that pushed her boobs together and up. Is that an okay bra for me to wear?

It is usually recommended for girls to wear age-appropriate bras during their pre-teen years. Bras worn by models are intended for older females, not young girls going through puberty.

Do girls' nipples get bigger with their breasts while going through puberty?

Girls' nipples grow proportionately to their bodies, so as their breasts grow, their nipples will grow.

What do nipples do?

Nipples are used for feeding a baby.

Why do boys have nipples?

Both girls and boys grow nipples because the same development of body parts occurs during the initial growth as an embryo in the mother's womb.

I have some kind of white stuff on my nipple. What is it?

The white stuff on the nipples is part of a natural fluid found in a girl's body. If a girl is concerned about this, or if a lot of fluid seems to be coming out of her nipple(s), she can ask a parent or other trusted adult to make an appointment for her to talk with a doctor.

My friend told me that her mom told her to feel her breasts every month. Why? It sounds strange that a girl has to feel herself up.

Once a girl's breasts begin to develop, it is a good idea for her to feel them to know what her breasts usually feel like and to check for anything unusual. Doing this is called breast self-examination (BSE) and is done once a month, generally after a girl has her period.

How do I do a breast self-exam?

To do breast self-examination, a girl raises one arm and gently pushes down on her breast area with her opposite hand to feel the area from under her armpit to her nipple. She then feels around her nipple in a circular manner. After checking one breast, the other breast is checked. This examination is done either lying down or standing up. Her doctor can also provide information about monthly breast examinations, including how to check for any lumps or irregularities.

If I find a lump in my boob, do I have cancer? My aunt had that and had surgery for it. Now I am scared.

Being diagnosed with breast cancer can be scary and sometimes it is difficult not to worry about something like this. Regarding lumps, many females have "cystic" lumps in their breasts that are a normal part of their bodies. However, when a cystic lump changes its shape or size, or if a new lump appears, a female should see her doctor for an examination. Her doctor may then recommend a particular procedure or test to check her breasts.

How can I prevent getting cancer?

There are things everyone can do to help prevent many diseases, including reducing the risk of getting cancer. They include:

- Exercising regularly to let the body move. By exercising, heart and respiration rates increase, bringing oxygen into the body.
- Eating nutritiously. People do not have to eat perfectly, yet should include fruit, vegetables, and whole grain foods into their eating plans.
- Watching stress levels. When feeling stressed, a person can practice relaxation exercises like yoga or meditation. Doing this helps to lower the chemical cortisol in the body. Exercise also helps to manage stress.
- Choosing to not use tobacco. Tobacco products have been proven to cause many health problems.
- Being aware of surrounding pollution. A cleaner environment helps to create healthier bodies.

Why are boys interested in boobs?

Some males say they like breasts because it is a natural instinct for males to like them. Some say they like breasts because they are there. No matter what the reason is, it is smart to be aware that many males like breasts.

Some of the boys in my class look at the girls' breasts and comment on them. Once they made fun of me because I did not have breasts yet (they called me pancake). Why do they do this?

Calling people names and commenting on their bodies are examples of harassing behavior. People who do these acts need to be taught they are inappropriate. Therefore, when any behavior like this happens, it needs to be reported to a trusted adult at school, like a teacher, counselor, or principal.

What is harassment?

Harassment is any intentional behavior making a person feel uncomfortable. For example, calling a person a name to make him or her feel bad or embarrassed is considered harassing behavior. While going through puberty, harassment includes saying hurtful comments about a person's changing body parts. If this happens, it needs to be reported to a trusted adult.

Why do some women show off their boobs, like by wearing certain shirts?

Some people feel comfortable showing more parts of their bodies than other people do. Yet this topic is tricky because people have the right to dress how they want, but certain outfits are not appropriate for school or work.

Will boys pay more attention to me if I show off my boobs?

Probably yes, but a girl is so much more than her breasts, and the attention may not be healthy. A girl should be respected for who she is and not for a part of her body.

Hairy Concerns for Girls

Where on a girl's body will she grow more hair during puberty?

During puberty, new darker hair grows in the armpit and private/pubic areas. Darker hair also grows on the legs of many girls.

Why do we get hair under our armpits?

A theory for why people grow armpit hair is the hair helps to lessen dampness when a person sweats and lowers the smell of sweat from the area.

At what age should you start shaving your armpits and legs?

When to start shaving depends upon a few things, including:

- if the girl's family or culture supports her shaving any hair,
- if the girl have enough hair to shave, and
- if the girl is mature enough to handle the responsibility of shaving.

If a girl has the support, hair, and maturity, she can most likely begin to shave.

Do I need to shave?

No. Shaving is a personal decision a girl should talk about with a parent or other trusted adult/puberty expert. In some cultures, girls do not shave at all or only shave certain parts of their bodies.

What things do I need to shave?

A girl needs a shaver, warm water, and shaving cream to shave. She may also use an electric shaver that does not require water or shaving cream.

Can I learn to shave on my own?

It is recommended a girl ask for help from a parent or trusted female puberty expert the first time she shaves to ensure she is cautious and does not hurt herself.

How do I shave my armpits and legs? Do I shave in a certain direction?

The overall steps for shaving these areas include:

1. Dampening the armpits and legs with warm water. Many females shave while taking a shower.
2. Placing shaving cream in the armpit areas and on areas of the legs to shave. Shaving cream can be placed on different body parts at separate times to avoid water washing it away.

3. For the armpit area, gently sliding the shaver at different angles (upwards, downwards, and sideways).
4. For the legs, gently sliding the shaver in an upward motion towards the knee, being extra careful around the ankles and knees.
5. After sliding the shaver one or two times, rinsing the shaver in water to remove the hair.
6. Continuing until all areas covered in shaving cream have been shaved.
7. Rinsing off all shaved areas with clean water and then patting them dry.

If I cut my legs from shaving, what do I do?

If a girl cuts her skin while shaving and the cut is only on the top layer of her skin, she can clean the area with soap and warm water, and then place a Band-Aid on it. Putting pressure on the area will also help to stop the bleeding. If the cut went deeper into the skin, the girl should tell/show a parent or other trusted adult in case she needs to go to a doctor's office for stitches.

Can I use soap to shave?

Shaving cream is made specifically for shaving in which it lessens the appearance of bumps on the skin afterwards. Some girls prefer to use soap, though, because shaving cream may be irritating to the skin.

How do I use an electric shaver?

Directions for using an electric shaver are found in or on the shaver's box/container. Basic instructions include charging the shaver, removing it from its stand, turning it on, and then gently rubbing it on the areas to be shaved. Water and shaving cream are not typically used with an electric shaver.

Where does hair grow in the vagina?

Pubic hair grows on the outer lips of a girl's vaginal opening, not in her vagina. And, as a girl gets older, pubic hair continues to grow a little up her front abdominal area and towards the lower edges of her "bikini" area.

What is the bikini area?

The bikini area is the front area located at the bottom of a bathing suit. For many girls, the pubic hair grows down their inner thighs and may stick out of the leg openings of a bathing suit or underwear. Some girls choose to remove or trim this hair.

Why do girls grow pubic hair?

Theories for why pubic hair grows include: the hair prevents germs from entering the three openings in the area; the hair keeps the genitals warm; and the hair deals with pheromones (smells that attract others).

Can you shave your private area?

Any hair can be shaved, but it is best to be taught how to do this. Therefore, before shaving her private area, a girl should talk with a parent or other trusted puberty expert.

Do girls have to remove their pubic hair?

No, girls do not have to remove their pubic hair. Many older girls trim their pubic hair when the hair seems to grow too much or gets "bushy" in the area. Others choose to remove pubic hair, yet they have to be very careful when doing this.

Do girls shave their arms?

Girls usually do not shave their arms.

I heard some women get body hair removed by waxing. Should I do this?

The decision to wax is personal and should be made with a parent or other trusted adult because a certified waxer who is specially trained to follow proper waxing procedures needs to be utilized. Also, anyone who chooses to get hair waxed needs to be aware that waxing could be painful, especially in sensitive areas.

I saw some hair removal products on television. Do these work?

Some people say the hair removal products advertised on television do work, but others say they do not work.

My sister goes to something with electricity to remove hair. Is she getting shocked?

Your sister is probably going to an electrolysis session to remove body hair. She is not getting shocked, although electrolysis does send a low-frequency form of electricity to the roots of the hair to help remove them. This procedure is usually not recommended for younger females.

Will I grow eyebrow hair?

When going through puberty, some girls might notice more hair in their eyebrow area. Hair has always been there, yet a girl can grow more or longer hair.

Can I get my eyebrows removed?

A person may choose to trim or tweeze some eyebrow hairs, yet does not usually remove all of them.

How do I tweeze my eyebrows?

It is best for a parent or other trusted adult/puberty expert to teach a girl how to tweeze her eyebrow hairs. The basic procedure, though, is to grab one hair at a time with a tweezer and pull it out in the direction is it growing.

Does tweezing hurt?

Sometimes tweezing can cause momentary pain and make the eyes tear.

I saw these women removing eyebrow hairs by threads in the mall. Is this safe?

Threading is a procedure that uses a strong thread to pull out different hairs in the eyebrow area. It is considered safe.

Why does my friend (a girl) have a mustache?

Some girls have darker hair above their upper lips or in other facial areas. This occurs because of their heredity or different hormone levels.

My great aunt has a mustache. Is she really a man? She has boobs.

No, women who have darker facial hair are not men, yet have grown darker hair in their mustache and chin areas because of their genetics and hormone levels.

Do older women have to shave their face?

No, women with facial hair do not need to shave their face unless they want to. Some women in this situation talk with a specialist about how to cope or remove the hair in a different manner than shaving.

What's What in the Female Reproductive System

What is the private area?

The private area is the area covered by a person's underwear and includes the vulva, vagina, and buttocks for females.

Why is it called a private area?

This area is called private because it is private and usually covered. For some people even talking about this area of the body is very personal.

Why is this area called the pubic area?

The private area is also known as the pubic area because of the pubic bone located right under the skin of a person's lower abdomen. This area grows pubic hair during puberty.

What is the reproductive system?

The reproductive system includes the body parts needed to create a baby. For girls, the system includes the vagina, uterus, ovaries, and Fallopian tubes. For boys, the system includes the testicles, scrotum, and penis. There are other parts in both of the systems, yet these are the commonly known parts.

What are the genitals for girls?

For girls, the external genitals include the vagina, labium, and clitoris. Some people refer to these parts as a girl's vulva.

What is a labia?

The labium (plural form of labia) are located in the opening area of the vagina and consist of outer and inner "lips" on both sides.

What are different names for the area "down there"?

Different phrases used for the reproductive system include the private area, pubic area, and genitals. There are also slang phrases like "your junk" or "your business."

How many openings does a girl have?

A girl has three openings located in her private area: the urethra (where urine/pee comes out); the vagina (where the menstrual fluid and babies come out); and the rectum (where feces or "poop" comes out).

Which hole is which in a girl's private area?

To understand which part is which, a girl can look at her private area with a mirror as she squats or lies on her back with her legs apart. What she will see from her top (abdomen) side of her body to her backside is:

1. The urethra: a small opening for urine, or pee, to leave the body.
2. The vagina: a bigger opening where the menstrual fluid is released.
3. The rectum: an opening for feces, or "poop," to leave the body.

How big is a girl's uterus?

A girl's uterus is approximately the size of her fist, but flat. Her uterus can expand to hold menstrual fluid and, if pregnant, a baby.

Why does the female reproductive system look like a moose's head?

An outline of the female's reproductive system may seem to look this way because the uterus, Fallopian tubes, and fimbria form an outline similar to one of a moose's head.

A teacher told us at school that talking about private parts to others may be considered harassment. What is that?

Harassment is any intentional behavior used to make a person or group of people feel uncomfortable. So when a person talks about particular topics, such as reproductive systems and puberty, but is asked to stop talking, it is best for the conversation to stop. If the person continues to talk about a sensitive topic, he/she should be reported for harassment. A person should also stop talking about sensitive topics if he/she notices the other person(s) becoming upset or uncomfortable.

Ovaries, Eggs, and Ovulation, Oh My!

How many ovaries does a girl have?
Girls are usually born with two ovaries.

Are girls ever born with one ovary?
Yes, a girl can be born with one ovary which can supply the eggs she needs for her menstrual cycle.

How big is an ovary?
An ovary is about the size and shape of an almond.

How big is an egg?
An egg is about one-tenth the size of a poppy seed.

How many eggs does a girl have?
A girl usually has between one million and two million eggs in her ovaries at birth. This amount goes down by the time she reaches puberty.

How does an egg form? How does a girl's egg get big?
When a girl is born, immature eggs are already in her ovaries. Upon reaching puberty, the eggs begin to mature.

How many eggs come out at a time?
One egg is usually released from one ovary per monthly menstrual cycle.

Does it matter what ovary the egg comes from?
No, either ovary can release an egg.

Can two eggs come out from the same ovary?
Yes, two eggs can come from the same ovary during a menstrual cycle. If these two eggs become fertilized, fraternal twins are created.

How long does it take an egg to go all the way?

A girl's menstrual cycle takes on average about twenty-eight days. After an egg is released from the ovary, it travels for about fourteen days to reach the uterine wall. If the egg is unfertilized, it will be removed with the menstrual fluid in the next few weeks.

Do girls have eggs forever or only at puberty?

Girls have eggs in their ovaries their whole lives unless they are surgically removed. Eggs are only released, though, when they have menstrual cycles.

What is this Discharge?

What is the white stuff on the inside of my underwear?

The whitish or clear fluid found on the inside of a girl's underwear is called a discharge.

What is a discharge?

Vaginal discharge is a body fluid that naturally comes out of a girl's vaginal opening. It is most noticeable two weeks before she gets her period. At this time, a girl may wipe her vaginal area after urinating and notice a "slippery" fluid or she may find fluid on the inside of her underwear.

How much later will you get your first period after your first discharge?

Many girls get a discharge from their vaginal opening about six months before their first period.

Can you have a discharge before your period?

Yes, many girls notice having a discharge about two weeks before getting their period.

Why do women get discharges before their periods?

Having a discharge usually means a girl is ovulating (an ovary has released an egg), in which the discharge helps the released egg travel towards the uterus. It can also help sperm travel to the released egg.

Should I be scared about having a discharge?

No, a girl should not be scared because the discharge is a natural occurrence for her body depending upon where she is in her menstrual cycle.

What can I do if I do not want discharge on my underwear?

A girl can wear a pantiliner on the inside of her underwear to collect discharge. This liner needs to be changed every three to four hours.

Should I go to a doctor if I have a discharge?

Having a discharge is part of a girl's menstrual cycle and does not require medical attention. Yet a girl should go to doctor if:

- the discharge has a weird or "yucky" smell;
- the discharge is grayish in color;
- the discharge looks like cottage cheese;
- along with a discharge, the vaginal area is sore or hurts; or
- she feels pain when she urinates (pees).

Why do I get a lot of discharge?

How much discharge a girl has depends upon her body, including her hormone levels and dietary habits. If a girl is concerned about having a lot of discharge, she can talk with a doctor, yet the amount might be normal for her body.

Your Monthly Visitor (Periods)

What is a period?

The word period is typically used to note a girl is menstruating, in which she "has her period."

What is menstruation? What is menstruating?

Menstruation occurs when a girl's uterus sheds the menstrual fluid/lining from her body. This fluid/lining exits from her vaginal opening and will look bloody.

What is the difference between menstrual fluid and menstrual lining?

For most people, the menstrual fluid and menstrual lining is the same thing. Specifically, the lining refers to the layer of cells which forms on the inside of the uterus during a female's menstrual cycle, and the fluid is what is released which includes the lining cells.

What are other names for having a period?

Other phrases include "being on the rag," "Aunt Sally is in town," and "Aunt Flo."

Why do girls make such a big deal over their period and use code names like "Tom" or "Aunt Flo"?

Code names, or slang terms, have been around for a long time. Sometimes girls feel more comfortable saying another term or phrase instead of saying the word period or menstruation. Also, some people were never taught the proper medical terms for certain body functions.

What does menarche mean?

Menarche is the term used for a girl's first period.

Normally at what age do girls get their period? What is the most common age for a girl to get her period?

The average age for girls to get their first period is twelve, yet girls can get their first period as early as eight years old or as late as sixteen years old.

Do you have your period in the fourth or fifth grade?

Some girls begin having their periods (menstrual cycle) in the fourth or fifth grade.

Does a girl get monthly periods right away?

When a girl begins menstruating, her periods are usually not on a monthly schedule. For example, her first period (menarche) might occur in August, and then her second period in November or December of the same year. After her body reaches a certain level of physical maturity, her period typically occurs monthly.

Is it true that you get your period when your mom did?

A girl may get her first period (menarche) at the same age as when her mother did, yet this is not always the case. Due to changes in diets and living conditions, the age of menarche (first period) depends upon each girl's body.

Is it true that thinner girls get their periods later?

Girls get their periods when their bodies mature to a point to experience periods. Some research has found girls who are heavier may be more likely to start their periods earlier, yet there are many factors to consider for what causes a girl to start menstruating.

How does the menstrual cycle (period) work?

The basics of the menstrual cycle include:

- The cycle lasts from the first day of a period (the first day of menstrual fluid release) until the day of a girl's next period. For example: If Lori gets her period on August 18th and then again on September 15th, her cycle lasted twenty-eight (28) days.
- A cycle can last anywhere from twenty-one to thirty-four (21 to 34) days once the girl becomes an older teen and adult. The typical amount of time for a cycle is twenty- eight (28) days, yet this varies for each girl.
- During the first days of a menstrual cycle, menstrual fluid, which includes blood, tissue, and an unfertilized egg, comes out of the girl's vaginal opening. These days are referred to having a period and typically lasts from two to seven days.
- After the menstrual fluid stops being released, certain hormones rise in the girl's body. These hormones send messages to the uterus to start forming another lining to prepare for the release of the next egg from an ovary. Also at this time, an ovary prepares to release a mature egg.
- About halfway into the cycle, the egg is released from the ovary and travels through a Fallopian tube to the uterus. This process takes a few days and is called ovulation. As this happens, the body

continues to send blood to the uterus. Sometimes a girl may feel some discomfort or mild cramping during ovulation.

- Upon not being pregnant, the girl's body prepares to release the newly collected menstrual fluid. At this point, the uterus stops collecting blood for its lining and releases the fluid with the unfertilized egg.

This whole process is called a cycle because it occurs about every month in a regular pattern.

How long does a period last? How long does it bleed for until it stops?

The length of a period ranges from two to seven days. This length can change each month, though, due to diet, exercise, sleep, and stress levels, as well as if a girl takes certain medications.

How much blood and other fluids come out the first time?

How much menstrual fluid is released during a girl's first period depends on the girl and can range from a few teaspoons to a few tablespoons.

How much blood usually comes out?

Over the two to seven days of a girl's period, about two to three tablespoons of blood come out. There are other fluids also released which increases this amount to about a half of a cup of overall fluid each menstrual cycle.

What is the "lighter" time of your period?

During the first days of a girl's period, more menstrual fluid usually comes out and is often referred to as the "heaviest" time of a period. Towards the end of a girl's period, less menstrual fluid comes out and is referred to the "lighter" time.

Should I feel scared about getting my period?

No, a girl does not need to feel scared about getting her period. Getting a period is a natural part of growing up and becoming a woman.

Why do you get your period? What is the purpose? Is there a reason? Why does your vagina bleed?

A girl gets a period to release her menstrual fluid which is a natural part of becoming a woman.

But why?

So one day, if a female chooses, she can have a baby. To create a baby, an egg needs to be released from a female's ovary and a menstrual lining needs to be formed.

Why does blood go to our uterus?

Blood travels to the uterus because it carries oxygen and nutrients allowing a fertilized egg to grow. When a female is not pregnant (her egg is unfertilized), this blood is released as her menstrual period. When a female is pregnant, this fluid helps supply oxygen and nutrients to the growing baby.

When you get your period, does the egg turn to blood?

No, the egg does not turn into blood.

Can I see a released egg in the blood?

No, a released egg is too small to see with the human eye.

Do you stop growing when you get your period?

No, a girl will continue growing taller and wider after getting her first period. This overall growth will stop when her body has grown to the size (a woman's size) it was meant to be.

What if a girl doesn't get her period?

If a girl does not get her period by the time she has reached her sixteenth birthday, it is advisable she speak with a doctor. The doctor will then check to see if she is maturing at a later age than other girls.

With your period, is there anything else besides bleeding?

The period is the bleeding part (release of fluids) of the menstrual cycle. Right before or during this time, a girl may feel some bloating in her abdominal area, breast tenderness, or moodiness. Some girls also experience cramping in the abdominal (belly) area.

How does it feel to have your period?

How a period feels depends upon the girl and her monthly cycle. Sometimes a girl has her period, yet does not feel any differently. Other months she may feel more tired or moody, or feel cramping in her lower abdominal (belly) area.

Does it hurt when girls get their periods?

Some girls feel cramping in their lower abdominal (belly) area right before or upon getting their periods. This cramping occurs because chemicals called prostaglandins are released making the uterus contract to push out the menstrual fluid.

What do cramps feel like?

Cramps feel like pressure or pain in the lower abdominal (belly) area.

Every couple of months I get a cramp near my uterus. Does this mean I'm getting my period?

Feeling a cramp in the lower abdomen could mean a girl is about to get her period or that an egg was released from an ovary (ovulation). This cramping feeling could also be a symptom of a stomach ache or gas pains.

Does the blood just squirt out or flow out?

Menstruation is a gradual process in which the menstrual fluid does not squirt out of a girl, yet slowly comes out.

My mom said that the second day of your period is the worst. Is that true?

It depends upon the female. Some girls feel the first day of their period is worse, some feel their second day is worse, and then other girls feel no particular day is the worst.

My mom told me to take a hot bath to stop cramps. How will a hot bath help?

A hot bath may help ease tense muscles which can lessen cramps. Yet, if her period is heavy, a girl might not feel she wants to take a bath. Instead, she can place a heating pad or hot water bottle on her lower abdomen to help ease any muscle tension.

Is there a way to get rid of your cramps?

Yes, there are many ways to get rid of cramps. Some forms of exercise may help ease them, including doing yoga or gentle stretches. Also, putting a heating pad or hot water bottle on the lower abdomen or taking medicine, like ibuprofen, with an adult's permission can help reduce the pain.

What is a heating pad?

A heating pad is a flat cushioned pad, about twelve by fifteen inches in size, which becomes hot when plugged into an electrical outlet and turned on. Usually, there are a variety of temperature settings on the heating pad.

What is a hot water bottle?

A hot water bottle is a bottle made of a flexible plastic material that holds hot or warm water.

I heard girls who live with other girls can get their periods at the same time. Is this true?

It is thought girls who live together unknowingly recognize the other girls' pheromones. This occurrence may enable girls to get their periods at the same time, yet there are many factors affecting girls' menstrual cycles.

What are pheromones?

Pheromones are natural chemicals released by animals, including people. Yet people are usually not aware of them because pheromones do not have a smell. Some people believe pheromones help people feel attracted to others.

Ready, Set, Go! Being Prepared for Your Period in Different Situations

What do you use when you have your period?
A girl typically uses either a pad or tampon when she has her period.

Which are better to use: menstrual pads or tampons? Do we use pads or just tampons? Are pads better for young girls? Are tampons better? Does it matter if you switch from a pad to a tampon?
Deciding to use a pad or tampon depends upon the girl, yet the majority of girls use pads when first getting their periods. When they are older, some use tampons or a combination of products.

What do you think is more comfortable: a pad or a tampon?
Using a pad or a tampon is a personal choice each girl has to make for herself, in which each girl needs to figure out what is most comfortable for her. What one girl chooses to use may be different from what another girl chooses.

Why are there pads and tampons with a smell?
Some pads and tampons are labeled as "scented" or "scented deodorant" because they have a smell added to them. Using these pads and tampons is a personal choice, and a girl should ask her doctor if scented products are a better choice for her.

What do I do with a used pad or tampon?
After removing a used pad or tampon, a girl wraps it in toilet paper and puts it into a garbage can. Many public women's restrooms have a small garbage can on the floor between stalls or on the wall of a stall to dispose of used pads and tampons, as well as applicators.

Do I throw a used pad or tampon into the toilet?
Throwing a pad or tampon into a toilet can cause plumbing problems, so it is advisable for a girl *to not* throw one into a toilet.

What do you do when your first period comes?

When a girl notices she has her period, she places a pad on the inside of her underwear or a tampon into her vaginal opening. If she is unsure of how to use a pad or tampon, she can talk with a parent or other trusted adult/puberty expert or follow the directions in/on the product packaging.

When you are in the shower, will your period just start bleeding?

No, a girl does not "just start bleeding" in the shower if she gets her period because the menstrual fluid does not quickly come out of a girl. Instead, she may notice bloody fluid appearing in the water as she rinses her vaginal area or on the towel after she dries the area.

Can I go swimming with my period? My friend told me I couldn't.

Yes, a girl can go swimming with her period. There are many girls who swim for exercise, are on swim teams, or who participate in triathlons. These girls swim regularly, including when they have their periods.

What happens when you are in the shower and you have your period?

When a girl has her period, she takes a shower as she usually does. She might choose to clean her vaginal area last, though, to rinse any fluid that may have slowly come out as she was showering. After drying herself off, she will place a pad onto her underwear or insert a tampon into her vaginal opening.

What do you do when you have your period on school days?

A girl still needs to go to school even if she has her period. On these days, she needs to bring pads or tampons to school for the day's use. Some girls also choose to bring an extra pair of underwear in case fluid leaks onto the underwear they are wearing.

What if I get my period during the school day?

If a girl gets her period and does not have a pad or tampon, she can put a little pile of toilet paper in the middle area of her underwear while in the bathroom. Then she should go to the nurse's office to get a pad because most schools have menstrual pads in the nurse's office for girls.

I am afraid that if I go to the nurse's office from the bathroom without asking my teacher first I will get into trouble. What should I do?

A girl might be afraid to go the nurse's office, but most nurses will help a girl by writing a pass or note to her teacher. These things happen and people usually understand.

What do you do if you get your period at school and the nurse is absent?

Even if the usual nurse is absent, a substitute nurse or office assistant can help a girl.

What do I do if my school does not have a nurse?

A girl can talk with a teacher, a teacher's aide, an office assistant, or anyone else she feels comfortable speaking with.

What if you get your period during school and people make fun of you? What should you do?

No one should make fun of a girl for getting her period or for anything else. Getting a period is natural for girls and anyone who makes fun of nature is being immature. So if a girl is being made fun of, the girl, or anyone witnessing this, needs to tell a trusted adult.

If you are at a sleepover and you get your period in the middle of the night, what should you do?

A girl can bring an extra pair of underwear and pads/tampons in case she gets her period at a sleepover. Underwear is usually changed every day, so having an extra pair of them is not noticeable. If a girl does not carry pads or tampons, she can ask her friend or her friend's parent where pads or tampons are kept. If she is nervous, the girl can call her parent or another trusted adult/puberty expert to ask for advice.

When you are at a friend's house and have your period but you don't want to ask an adult for a pad, what should you do?

Sometimes girls look in a bathroom cabinet for a pad, yet it is respectful to let the friend or the friend's parent know. A girl can also call home for help.

Why does everyone need to know about me getting my period?

No one needs to know when a girl has her period because having a period is personal and who a girl chooses to share this with is up to her. Yet some girls like to tell others because talking about it removes some fears or may clear up any questions or concerns.

What if someone asks you if you got your period and I don't want to tell them? What should you do?

If a girl wants to keep her period private, she can politely say, "I do not want to talk about this with you. If I change my mind, I will let you know." If the person continues to ask, she can tell him/her this again, and then walk away.

Say if I want to tell other girls that I have my period?

A girl can tell others she has gotten her period, yet she has to remember some people can keep a secret and other people cannot.

What do you do if you have a period and leak blood onto your pants?

If a girl leaks menstrual fluid onto her clothing, she can wrap a sweatshirt or sweater around her waist, so her bottom area is covered. If she has other clothing with her, she can change into them. The girl can also ask to call home for other clothing. Whatever she does, as long as the girl acts casually, no one will notice the situation, but if she panics, she is more likely to draw attention to herself.

What happens when you have your period and you are wearing white pants?

A girl can wear white pants when she has her period, yet she has to be careful about preventing menstrual fluid from leaking onto her underwear and white pants. If this happens, she can wrap a long sleeve shirt, sweater, or sweatshirt around her waist to cover her bottom area, and, as soon as she can, change into another outfit. Sometimes this kind of thing happens, and a girl needs to cope as best as possible.

What happens if someone "pants" you when you have your period? ("Pantsing" is a slang term meaning someone pulling down another person's pants.)

"Pantsing" is disrespectful and should not happen at all. If it does happen, the girl (or boy) needs to talk with a trusted adult immediately.

If I stain my underwear I have to throw them out, right?

If a girl gets stains from her menstrual period on her underwear, she needs to clean them. The stains may not be completely removed after cleaning, yet a girl can keep this underwear to wear during future periods. Many women admit to having a pair or two of clean yet stained underwear they wear during their periods.

How do I remove bloodstains from my clothing?

To remove bloodstains, soak the clothing in water as soon as possible. Sometimes putting salt into cold water as the clothing soaks helps, as well as rubbing laundry detergent directly onto the stain. There are also laundry stain removers a girl can use.

What should I do if only a man, like my dad, is around to help me?

A girl may feel awkward, yet she can ask her dad for help with her period. He might even suggest she talk with a female he trusts. If a girl feels uncomfortable talking with her dad, though, she can go to a trusted female puberty expert, like a teacher, coach, or older sister, because most females help other females with their periods.

Long or Short? Maxi or Mini? With or Without Wings? So Many Choices with Pads

What is a pad?

A pad is made of specific materials used to collect menstrual fluid. One side of the pad collects the fluid, and the other side has an adhesive strip to hold the pad in place onto the girl's underwear, between her legs.

When do you start using pads?

A girl starts using pads when she first gets her period.

How often do you change a pad?

How often a girl needs to change a pad will depend on how much menstrual fluid comes out, yet a recommended time to change a pad is every three to four hours.

What types of pads are there?

There are many types of pads to choose from including different sizes and absorbencies. What size to use is determined by what size the girl prefers and the size of her body. In regards to absorbency, many girls use more absorbent pads for the first days of their periods and then use pads with less absorbency as their periods become lighter.

What are pads with "wings"?

Pads with wings have additional absorbent material that is placed over the sides of a girl's underwear, sticking to its bottom side. "Wings" help stop leakages on the sides of a pad, and may limit stains on a girl's underwear caused by the menstrual fluid.

What is a pantiliner?

A pantiliner is a small, thin pad made of absorbent material and is worn in a girl's underwear when her period is lighter or when she has a discharge.

Is there such a thing as reusable pads for a girl's period?

Yes, there are reusable pads a girl can use during her period. These pads are washed after every use and need to be changed every three to four hours like regular pads.

Are there underpants with built in pads or pantiliners for periods?

Yes, there are underpants with built-in pads or pantiliners. These underpants are for lighter days of a girl's period or worn for additional protection with another product (for example, with tampons). These products can be bought at certain stores or online.

Which brand of pads should girls buy?

There are many brands of pads for girls to use and, although there are similarities between them, some are less expensive or have a particular feature. The choice of what brand to buy is personal and depends on the girl.

What if I am embarrassed about buying pads at the store?

There is no reason for a girl to be embarrassed when buying pads. Girls get periods and, therefore, need pads. To lower anxiety, though, a girl can shop with a friend or puberty expert and take some deep breaths. Buying pads does not take long, but the more a girl procrastinates, the more anxious she may become.

Do you wear a pad to sleep?

Yes, many girls wear pads while sleeping when they have their periods. There are longer pads made for sleeping, but if a girl does not have one, she wears a regular sized pad.

Do I have to change my pad in the middle of the night?

A girl can wear one pad as she is sleeping, yet if she wakes up in the middle of the night and needs or wants to change the pad, she can.

What do I do if I bleed onto my sheets or bed? Do they get thrown out?

If any menstrual fluid gets on a girl's sheets or mattress, they need to be cleaned.

How can I prevent staining my bed?

To prevent stains, a girl can place a towel or padded liner between her and her bottom sheet to collect any leaking menstrual fluid.

Can you get an infection by wearing a pad for too long?

Yes, a girl can get an infection by wearing a pad for too long. Also, wearing a pad for more than a few hours can create a "not so nice" smell other people may notice. Luckily, because girls urinate regularly and usually change their underwear every day, girls will most likely remember they are wearing a pad and, therefore, change them.

What if you go swimming, do you wear a pad? Can you swim with a pad on (when you have your period)?

Girls do not wear pads when swimming, yet wear tampons or menstrual cups. If a girl does not want to wear a tampon or menstrual cup and her menstrual flow is not heavy, she may choose to change into her bathing suit right before entering the water. Then, after swimming, she can change out of her bathing suit into clothing, placing a pad in her underwear.

"You Put It Where?" and Other Questions about Tampons

What is a tampon? What is the use of a tampon?

A tampon is made of absorbent material and is placed inside a girl's vaginal opening to absorb her menstrual fluid.

I heard some tampons have an applicator. What is that?

Most tampons come with a cardboard or plastic applicator to help place the actual tampon (absorbent material) into a girl's vaginal opening. This applicator consists of two tubes: a slimmer inner tube and a wider outer tube. The absorbent material is located in the wider tube with its string going through the slimmer tube, sticking out at its end.

Do tampons come with instructions?

Yes, instructions for how to correctly use tampons are provided either on the box of tampons or an insert. Most directions include diagrams to show their use.

How does a tampon go into a girl? How do you use tampons? How do you get a tampon in? You put it where?

First, a girl should wash her hands with soap and warm water. Then, to insert the tampon, she gently pushes the wider part of the applicator inside her vaginal opening, holding onto its base. Once it is inside her, she then pushes the inner tube into the wider tube. Doing this places the actual tampon into her vagina with the string of the tampon remaining at her vaginal opening. After the tampon is placed in all of the way, a girl removes the outer tube with the inner tube inside of it, throws it away, and then washes her hands again.

What should I do if using a tampon hurts or feels weird?

If a girl feels pain or "weird" when wearing a tampon, it may be because it was not placed into her vaginal opening all the way. To fix this, she can push the tampon in a little more with a clean finger. If it still hurts or feels weird, she should take out the tampon and talk with a parent or other trusted adult/puberty expert.

What do I do with the applicator? Do I throw the applicator into the toilet? What do I do with the tubes after the tampon is in?

After inserting the tampon into her vaginal opening, a girl places the applicator into a garbage can. Many public women's restrooms have a small garbage can on the floor between stalls or on the wall of a stall to dispose of applicators and used tampons and pads. A girl should *not* throw the applicator into the toilet because it can clog the pipes.

How often do I change a tampon?

A tampon should be changed every four to eight hours, depending upon the heaviness of the menstrual flow. It is advisable to not wear a tampon for more than eight hours.

How does a girl remove a tampon?

After cleaning her hands, a girl removes a tampon by gently pulling the tampon string out of her vaginal opening which will pull the tampon out.

What if the tampon string gets caught? How do you get the tampon out if the string disappears inside of her?

If a tampon's string slips into a girl's vaginal opening, she should:

1. wash her hands,
2. squat down towards the floor, or lay on her back with her legs open,
3. place a clean finger into the opening of her vagina,
4. feel for the tampon, including its string, and
5. gently pull it out.

Does it hurt when you remove a tampon from your body?

No, removing a tampon should not hurt. Yet, if a girl gets nervous, the muscles in her vaginal area may tighten, making it more difficult for the tampon to be removed. If this happens, the girl should take a few slow, deep breaths to relax, and then try to get the tampon out again.

Yuck, taking a tampon out sounds gross. Is it?

A girl's body is not gross, and it is natural for girls to have vaginas and periods. But if a girl feels uncomfortable about the use of tampons, she should not use them.

My mom told me that a girl needs to touch her vaginal area to find where to place a tampon. Isn't that considered gross?

No, a girl who touches her private area is not gross. And if a girl chooses to use tampons, a girl needs to know where to properly place them.

Will I ever have to use a tampon?

No, not all girls use tampons. This decision is an individual choice each girl makes.

Do tampons come in different sizes?

Yes, tampons come in different sizes, and girls should wear the size most comfortable for them or for particular days. Smaller or petite sized tampons are used for the lighter days of a girl's period or by girls who feel more comfortable wearing smaller tampons. Larger tampons are used during the heavier days of a girl's period.

Can I sleep with a tampon in my vagina?

Yes, a girl can sleep while wearing a tampon. As soon as she wakes up, the tampon needs to be changed/removed.

How do you pee if you're wearing a tampon?

Urine (pee) comes out of the urethra and, because a tampon is placed into a different opening, the vaginal opening, a girl can continue to wear her tampon while urinating.

If a girl urinates while wearing a tampon, does she still have to wipe herself?

Yes, a girl always needs to wipe her vaginal area after urinating to remove any drops of urine.

Can you get sick if you leave a tampon in too long?

Yes, a girl can get an infection if a tampon is kept in her vagina for too long due to the growth of unhealthy germs.

I heard some girls get hurt from tampons. Are they dangerous?

Toxic Shock Syndrome (TSS) was discovered years ago by some women who used tampons. TSS caused them to become sick. Today, according to the Food and Drug Administration (FDA), tampons are safer to use. A girl needs to change her tampon, though, every few hours, and use a tampon with the right amount of absorption she needs.

Other Curious Questions about Girls

When you get a pain in the vagina, what does it mean?

If a girl feels any pain, she needs to talk with a parent or other trusted adult/puberty expert. If her pain is in the lower abdominal (belly) area, it may be cramps. Cramps happen when a girl gets her period, even before menstrual fluid comes out. If a girl has pain because she fell on something in her vaginal area (like the middle bar of a bicycle) or something was placed at or in her vaginal opening, a parent or other trusted adult/puberty expert should have her talk with a doctor. The doctor will then figure out how to resolve any pain.

What does bloating mean?

Bloating occurs when the abdominal (belly) area of a girl feels swollen, making her feel bigger. This feeling is more common right before a girl gets her period, when she has her period, or during certain parts of puberty.

If I feel bloated, what should I do?

One way to get rid of feeling bloated is to exercise because exercising releases chemicals called endorphins that help people feel better, both emotionally and physically. Examples of exercising include practicing yoga postures, riding a bike, jogging, playing sports, and walking a dog.

When you get your period, does it smell? Does the blood smell?
The release of menstrual fluid during a girl's cycle can smell if a girl does not clean herself properly or does not change her pads/tampons regularly. Smells can also occur upon waking up in the morning or after exercising. When this happens, the girl should bathe and change her underwear and pad/tampon. If the smells do not disappear after washing and changing, she should talk with a parent or other trusted adult/puberty expert to make an appointment with a doctor to ensure she does not have an infection.

Why is your period so gross?
Periods occur because a girl's body goes through the natural process of her uterus cleaning itself out once a month. This process may seem gross, but it is part of being a pubescent girl and becoming a woman.

Do periods affect the way you act?
Sometimes periods affect how girls act. Some girls act older because, once they get their periods, they feel older. Some girls act sillier because they are nervous about their bodies changing. And some girls are moodier because of the changes in body hormones.

I was in a health food store and walked by the area with tampons and pads. I saw something like a plastic cup in a box for girls to use with their periods. What is this?
This "cup" is another product a girl can use when she has her period. The "cup" looks like a little cup, is made of flexible material, and is placed into the vagina to collect the menstrual fluid.

Do you reuse this "cup"?
Yes, a girl reuses this cup during her period after it is cleaned.

How do you wear this "cup"?
A girl needs to insert the cup into her vaginal opening in a particular manner. Detailed directions for how to do this are explained and shown on the box or insert of the product, as well as on the internet.

Can you share this "cup"?

No, girls should not share a menstrual "cup." Sharing anything that touches body fluids shares germs that can cause diseases.

I heard a girl say that she douches when she has her period. What is it? Is it safe?

A douche is a product used to flush away vaginal fluids from the vagina. Douching is *not* recommended unless under the supervision of a doctor because it removes healthy bacteria living in the vagina and increases the chances of an infection.

Why do you douche before you have your period?

A girl does not douche before, during, or after her period. Most doctors believe douching is never needed unless a girl has an infection requiring a particular type of douche.

When you get your period will you have a baby?

No, a girl will only have a baby when a male's sperm fertilizes one of her eggs. So once a girl starts getting her period, she can become pregnant if she engages in sexual behaviors (has sex). Pregnancy can also occur during the time right before her first menstrual period.

Do you get more pimples during your period?

Some girls will get pimples right before or during their period because of the release of hormones during the menstrual cycle. To prevent pimples from happening, girls should wash their face with warm water and soap a few times a day and try not to touch their face with dirty hands.

Do boys have periods? Why won't boys bleed? Why do girls have periods and boys don't?

No, boys do not have periods because they do not have uteruses, eggs, or menstrual fluid.

Do animals (female animals) have periods?

Some female animals have something like a period. For example, a female dog goes into "heat" once or twice a year, which means the dog will have a bloody discharge from her vulva area for a period of time.

If my period lasts for over a week, should I be worried?

Some girls experience longer periods than other girls. If a girl has her period longer than a week, though, she should talk with a doctor to ease her worries and have her hormone levels checked.

Do you get a period throughout your whole life? Do people ever stop having their period? When does it end? Is it true you have periods until age fifty-five? Your period stops when you are fifty, right? When you're older, does your period go away? When do periods stop? (This question is asked in a variety of ways.)

A female has a menstrual cycle from puberty until menopause. The menstrual cycle also stops temporarily when a woman becomes pregnant, then resumes after the baby is born.

What is menopause?

Menopause occurs when a woman stops getting her period and her ovaries stop releasing eggs because of a change in hormone levels.

At what age is menopause?

Menopause occurs for some women in their forties, yet most women experience menopause during their fifties.

When your period ends (you stop getting it), can you still have a baby?

Once her menstrual cycle ends, a woman is unable to have a baby unless a particular procedure is done.

Do boys have menopause too?

Men do not go through a female-type menopause, yet experience other body changes as they age.

How many periods does a girl have in her life?

How many periods a girl has in her life will depend upon when she first starts getting her period and when they stop. For example: If Lori began her monthly period at the age of thirteen, and gets her period almost regularly once a month until the age of fifty-three, she will have her period (twelve times forty) approximately four hundred and eighty (480) times in her lifetime.

Why does your vagina tickle when you watch inappropriate things?

The "tickle" feeling, or nice tingly feeling, is the body's natural way of telling a girl she is "turned on" or sexually excited. This feeling can also happen when a girl talks to or sees a person she likes.

Is it possible for a girl to get an erection? If yes, where? Guys get boners. What happens to girls?

When boys are sexually excited, blood rushes to their penis making it firm and larger. A nickname for this is "boner." Girls also have a response when they are sexually excited. This response includes the creation of a slippery fluid in the girl's vaginal opening, her vaginal lips (labium) becoming swollen and redder in color, her clitoris getting a little larger and sticking out a bit further, and the girl feeling pleasant tingling sensations in the area.

What is a clitoris?

The clitoris is a small sensitive organ located towards the top fold of a girl's vaginal opening. If a girl lies on her back, the clitoris is seen or felt at the top of her labia lips, also known as the inner fold of her vulva.

Prepping Reminders

Both girls and boys are curious about the changes girls experience during puberty. Therefore, topics you can choose to prep for include:

- the changing of a girl's body shape, including breast development and widening of hips;
- new hair growth in the armpit, leg, and pubic areas;
- the maturing of reproductive parts;
- the beginning of ovulation and menstruation; and
- decision making about menstrual products.

Questions about Boys

The following questions are written in the manner of how children ask about situations pertaining to boys. Some questions may seem to be repeated, yet the author desires parents to understand the variety of ways children can ask the same question. Most spelling is correct, yet some errors are left to demonstrate how children sometimes misspell or mispronounce words.

Growth Spurts

When do boys start to go through puberty?
Most boys begin puberty between the ages of nine and fourteen.

How do guys know when they have reached puberty?
Boys know they are going through puberty when they notice a smelly body odor, hair growth in new places, weight gain, a growth spurt in height, acne, and/or a changing voice. They also notice their penis and testicles becoming larger in size.

When will I grow taller?
A boy begins to grow taller when certain hormones are released and his body receives messages from his brain telling the body to grow.

How can I grow taller faster?
A boy may want to grow taller at an earlier age, yet has to be patient with his body because it will grow at the speed it is meant to grow.

I am the shortest boy in my class. Will I always be that way?

No, sometimes the boy who is the last to start growing taller ends up being the tallest. This occurrence will depend, though, upon the boy's body as well as his peers' bodies.

Why do a boy's shoulders get bigger?

Upon reaching a certain age, the hormone testosterone increases to a higher level enabling a boy's body to grow into a man's body. This growth includes the broadening of his shoulders.

Does a boy's butt grow during puberty?

When growing into an adult sized body, every part of the boy's body grows, including his buttocks, making his body proportional.

Why don't men get breasts?

Girls develop breasts because they have more of the hormones estrogen and progesterone that are needed to develop breasts. Boys have less of these hormones and, therefore, do not develop breasts. Yet boys can develop fatty tissue in their chest area.

My doctor said that having breast tissue during puberty is normal for some boys. Is that true?

Yes, some boys have noticeable tissue in their chest area during puberty. As they continue to go through puberty, this tissue usually disappears.

If I am heavy will I have boobs? I saw a man on the beach with big breasts, and he was also really big. Is that normal?

Many heavier males have more fatty tissue in their chest area, yet they do not grow breasts like females.

I heard of boys growing big breasts and needing them removed. What is that?

Some boys have a condition called gynecomastia, which is the growth of excess tissue in the chest area. When this occurs, a boy can talk to a doctor about possible treatments.

Can a man with a fatty chest feed a baby?
No, a man cannot feed a baby with his chest or nipples, but he can feed a baby with a baby bottle (holding one for a baby).

How can a man get rid of his "man boobs"?
Exercise, including aerobic exercises and strength training, is one way to lose excess fatty tissue and tone the body.

Do, Re, Mi, Fa, So, Laaaaaaaaaaaaaaaa! (Voice Changes)

Why do boys get a deeper voice?
As a boy goes through puberty, his larynx, also known as the voice box, grows larger and thicker. This growth also creates a deeper voice because the vocal cords in the voice box stretch like rubber bands producing a change of sound while talking.

Why does my voice squeak sometimes? How come my voice sometimes cracks?
As a boy's larynx grows, so does his vocal cords and facial bones. This growth process requires a few months, in which a boy's voice may crack or make "squeaking" sounds during this time. It may be embarrassing, but he will outgrow this stage.

Sometimes when I answer the phone, people think I am my mom or a girl. Why?
When answering a phone, a boy may be mistaken for a girl or a woman because his larynx is growing making his voice become higher pitched at times. A more mature voice develops after reaching a certain point in puberty, making him sound like a man when answering the phone.

Is the Adam's apple a bone in your neck?
Yes, the Adam's apple is the larynx bone. When the Adam's apple grows, it changes its position, making it stick out from the throat. Some boys have this bone sticking out more than others, making it more noticeable.

Do girls have Adam's apples?

Yes, girls have Adam's apples, yet they are not as noticeable because they do not grow as much as boys' Adam's apples grow.

Hairy Concerns for Boys

Where do boys grow hair during puberty?

Boys begin to grow hair in their armpit, chest, facial, and pubic areas. For some boys, their leg and arm hair grow darker and thicker.

When do boys grow armpit hair? When should boys start getting hair on their armpits and penis? When do boys grow pubes?

Just like other changes at puberty, the growth of new or darker hair depends upon the boy. Some boys begin to grow new or darker hair in places as early as nine years old while others experience this growth at ages eleven, twelve, and thirteen.

Can you start to grow a mustache in the first grade and when you are older?

A boy may grow a mustache upon reaching a certain point of puberty. At first, a few facial hairs appear on his chin and cheeks and then under his nose. This facial hair growth is not typical when a boy is in the first grade, yet occurs most often when a boy is in the seventh, eighth, or ninth grade.

Will I be able to grow a beard and mustache?

All boys grow facial hair, yet some boys grow more hair than others. This difference means that not all boys will be able to grow a full beard and mustache covering all lower parts of the face with the same amount of hair.

At what age should you start shaving your face?

When to start shaving depends upon a few things, including:

- if the boy's family or culture supports him shaving any hair,
- if the boy has enough hair to shave, and
- if the boy is mature enough to handle the responsibility of shaving.

If a boy has the support, hair, and maturity, he can most likely begin to shave.

What things do I need to shave?
A boy needs a shaver, warm water, and shaving cream to shave. Or he can use an electric shaver that does not typically require water or shaving cream.

Can I use soap to shave instead of shaving cream?
Shaving cream is made specifically for shaving in which it lessens the appearance of bumps on the skin afterwards. Some males prefer to use soap, though, because shaving cream may be irritating to the skin.

Can I use someone else's shaver?
It is healthier for a boy to use his own shaver because sharing a shaver passes germs.

Do I shave in a certain direction?
Many men recommend shaving in the same direction of the growing hair, which is typically in the direction towards the chin.

How do I learn to shave my face?
A boy can ask a parent or other trusted adult/puberty expert to demonstrate how to shave his face so he can learn how to be cautious and not hurt himself. This person can also help him get his own shaver.

Can I learn to shave on my own?
It is recommended a boy ask for help from a parent or trusted male puberty expert the first time he shaves to ensure he is cautious and does not hurt himself.

How do I shave my face?
The overall steps for shaving the face and neck include:

1. Dampening the face and neck with warm water.
2. Placing shaving cream on all parts of the face and neck to be shaved.

3. For the face, gently sliding the shaver in a downward fashion, towards the mouth/chin.
4. For the neck, gently sliding the shaver in an upward motion towards the chin.
5. After one or two slides with the shaver, rinsing the shaver in water. Many boys put water into a sink to rinse their shaver.
6. Continuing to shave until all areas covered in shaving cream are shaved.
7. Rinsing off all shaved areas with clean water, and then patting them dry with a clean towel.

Why do I see men put toilet paper on their faces when they bleed?

Sometimes a man cuts or "nicks" his skin as he shaves. To help stop the bleeding, some men place a tissue of some sort, like a small piece of toilet paper, onto the cut. There is a variety of ways, though, to stop the bleeding and clean the cut.

How would I use an electric shaver?

Directions for using an electric shaver are in/on its box/container. Basic instructions include charging the shaver, removing it from its stand, turning it on, and then gently rubbing it on the areas to be shaved. Shaving cream and water are not typically used with electric shavers.

Why do many male athletes shave their body hair?

Some athletes shave their body hair because it reduces drag when competing in sports, like swimming and road bike racing.

Do I have to shave my chest hair?

Although there has been an increase of this habit by some males, there is no need for males to shave or remove their chest hair. For those who do shave this area, they need to realize that whatever hair is shaved grows back as "stubble," which may feel uncomfortable for a day or so.

What is "stubble"?

Stubble is the term used for hair growing again after being shaved. When this happens, the skin area feels rough, like sandpaper.

Do you shave your chest the same way you shave your face?

Yes, a male would shave his chest in a similar manner as his face. He can either use shaving cream, warm water, and a shaver or an electric shaver. If using a non-electric shaver, the direction of the strokes will vary depending on the area being shaved.

How quickly will my hair grow in again after I shave?

How quickly a boy's hair grows depends upon his body. Some boys will not have stubble on their face for a day or more after shaving, while other boys will have hair grow in a few hours after shaving.

What is a "five o'clock shadow"?

A "five o'clock shadow" is the phrase used by men when their facial hair begins to grow back later in the day. Even though they shaved earlier in the day, around five o'clock in the evening a dark stubble or shadow appears.

Why do guys penises get hairy? Why/how do we get hair on our testicles?

Hair does not grow on a boy's penis, but in the area around his penis and on his scrotum (the pouch of skin holding the testicles). One theory for why boys grow pubic hair is the hair helps to keep the area warm in cold weather and protected from sweat and germs.

In Germany, boys shave their penis and armpit hair. Is that normal?

What hair to remove is a personal choice and people living in different places of the world remove different body hair. Because it is uncommon in America, a boy may think this is strange, but it is just a different cultural custom.

Will boys' eyebrows grow eventually?

Yes, boys will grow more hair in their eyebrow areas with some growing more eyebrow hair than others.

How come my grandfather has weird eyebrows? Why does my granddad have hair growing out of his ears?

As a man ages, his eyebrow, ear, and nose hair continue to grow, becoming longer. These areas can be trimmed with special scissors or hair trimmers.

How come some men get bald, but grow longer eyebrow, nose, and ear hairs? Can't that hair go to the top of their heads instead?
A man cannot control where his hair grows as he ages. Losing hair in some places and gaining hair in other places is a natural occurrence for both males and females.

Can a man get a hair transplant if he is losing hair?
Yes, some people who are going bald or have thinning hair may choose to get a procedure done for the hair on their heads to look fuller. Doing this is a personal decision and requires time and money.

What's What in the Male Reproductive System

What is the private area? Do men have two privates: the penis and the testicles?
The private area is the area covered by a boy's underwear and includes the boy's penis, scrotum, testicles, and buttocks.

Why is it called a private area?
This area is called the private area because it is private. Talking about this area of the body is personal to many people.

Why is this area called the pubic area?
This area is called the pubic area because of the pubic bone located right under the skin of a person's lower abdomen. This area gets covered with pubic hair at some point during puberty.

Isn't this area called the public area?
No, this area is called the pubic area and, in the United States, is not usually shown in public.

What is the reproductive system?
The reproductive system includes the body parts needed to create a baby. For boys, the system includes the testicles, scrotum, and penis. For girls, the system includes the vagina, uterus, Fallopian tubes, and ovaries. There are other parts in both of the systems, yet these are the commonly known parts.

What are the genitals for boys?

For boys, the genitals include the penis, testicles, and scrotum.

What are all of the different names for the area "down there"?

The different names for "down there" include the private area, pubic area, genitals, reproductive system, and the slang term "your junk."

A teacher told us at school that talking about private parts to others may be considered harassment. What is that?

Harassment is any intentional behavior used to make a person or group of people feel uncomfortable. So when a person talks about particular topics, such as reproductive systems and puberty, but is asked to stop talking, it is best for the conversation to stop. If the person continues to talk about a sensitive topic, he/she can be reported for harassment. A person can also stop talking about sensitive topics if he/she notices the other person(s) becoming upset or uncomfortable.

How's it Hanging? Down and to the Left (Testicles and the Scrotum)

What is a testicle?

A testicle is a round gland found in a boy's scrotum.

Are testicles "nuts"?

"Nuts" is a slang term for testicles. "Balls" is another slang term.

What do the boys' balls do?

Testicles release testosterone and produce, then store, sperm.

What is the "bag" that holds the testicles?

The "bag" or sac is called a scrotum and is located behind the boy's penis.

Why do your testicles grow larger?

The testicles and scrotum grow larger during puberty to become proportional to a boy's growing body.

Are testicles the same size?

No, one testicle is usually larger than the other. Just like a boy's hands are not exactly the same size and shape, neither are his testicles.

Why do a boy's testicles hang outside his body? Why aren't testicles inside the body like a girl's ovaries?

Because sperm need a slightly cooler temperature than a boy's internal temperature, the testicles hang outside his body allowing them to be a little cooler.

Why is one testicle lower than the other?

A theory for why one testicle typically hangs lower than the other one includes it minimizes friction or discomfort for a boy and allows for a cooler temperature around each testicle.

How many testicles should a boy have?

The majority of boys are born with two testicles, although only one is needed to make testosterone and sperm.

Can a boy be born with only one testicle?

Yes, a boy can be born with only one testicle.

Can a boy be born with three or more testicles? Can a boy be born with three balls in his penis?

Yes, a boy can be born with three testicles, although this is a rare occurrence.

What happens when a boy is born with three testicles?

If a boy is born with three testicles, what will happen depends on the location of the additional testicle. Upon it being discovered, a doctor will check to see if the third testicle impairs or disturbs any bodily function or causes discomfort. If necessary, one testicle may be surgically removed. If it is not necessary to be removed, the third testicle will be monitored.

Could you live without testicles? Is it possible to have no nuts or balls?

Yes, it is possible for a boy to have no testicles.

I heard about some famous men who had a disease in their testicles. What disease did they have?

Some years ago, comedian Tom Green and former cyclist Lance Armstrong announced to the public they were battling cancer, including testicular cancer (cancer of a testicle). Both men had one of their testicles, the cancerous one, removed.

Is a man still a man with one testicle?

Yes, a man with one testicle is a man.

How can I prevent getting cancer?

There are things everyone can do to help prevent many diseases, including reducing the risk of getting cancer. They include:

- Exercising regularly to let the body move. By exercising, heart and respiration rates increase, bringing oxygen into the body.
- Eating nutritiously. People do not have to eat perfectly, yet should include fruit, vegetables, and whole grain foods into their eating plans.
- Watching stress levels. When feeling stressed, a person can practice relaxation exercises like yoga or meditation. Doing this helps to lower the chemical cortisol in the body. Exercise also helps to manage stress.
- Choosing to not use tobacco products. Tobacco products have been proven to cause many health problems.
- Being aware of surrounding pollution. A cleaner environment helps to create healthier bodies.

The Penis- The Long and Short of It

What is a "peanes"/penis? What is a "dick"?

Penis is the proper medical term used to refer to the boy's genital that releases urine and semen.

What are slang terms for penis?

Slang terms for penis include "dick," "wiener," "pee hose," "wee-wee," "pee-pee," "cock," and "the snake."

Why are there so many slang terms for the penis?

Some people say slang terms because they were never taught the proper medical terms when they were younger. Also, sometimes people make up or use slang terms to make others laugh. Yet people have to be careful of what terms they use because slang terms can be offensive to some people.

What is the tube that the body fluids in the penis come out of?

The tube that removes both urine and semen from a boy's body is called a urethra.

My dad told me that when I was born, I was circumcised. What is this?

A circumcision is the cutting of the skin on the tip of a boy's penis (foreskin) to allow the skin to spread out over the top of his penis.

How come some boys are circumcised and others aren't?

The decision to have a boy's penis circumcised is usually made by the boy's family after he is born. His religion and culture typically influences this decision. If a boy is uncircumcised when he is younger, he can decide to have the procedure done later in his life.

Is it bad if a boy doesn't have a circumcision?

It is not bad if a boy's penis is uncircumcised. A difference, though, is that he needs to clean the area beneath his foreskin (the glans).

Does a circumcision hurt the baby boy?

Due to the foreskin area having numerous nerve endings, pain most likely occurs during a circumcision. Doctors attempt to lower any pain, though, by providing numbing medication before and after the procedure.

Is it bad if I want to talk about my penis?

Whether it is appropriate to talk about a penis or other reproductive parts depends on the situation and location. If a boy is asking his doctor questions, it is appropriate because doctors are supposed to answer questions dealing with the body. But if a boy wants to talk with others about his or other people's reproductive parts, both the boy and the other people need to feel comfortable with the discussion.

When should I not talk about my penis?

There are definite inappropriate times and places for talking about reproductive parts. Examples include during a math lesson, in the common areas of school where others can overhear the conversation (like in hallways, by lockers, or in the cafeteria), or when the person knows the conversation embarrasses other people.

Why does it hurt when I get hit in the penis?

Being hit in the penis hurts because there are many nerve endings in a boy's penis and the surrounding areas, making it sensitive. When a boy gets hit there, the nerve endings feel it and register the feeling as pain.

If you get hit in the penis, will it affect your babies?

If a boy gets hit in his penile area and the penis is damaged, it may impact future baby making possibilities. There would have to be significant damage, though. To ensure he is fine, a boy who is hit in his penile area should talk with a parent or other trusted adult in case he needs to see a doctor to be checked.

How do I prevent getting hit in the penis?

A boy can prevent being hit in his penile area by:

- wearing a sports cup when playing sports;
- being careful when stopping on a bike (hitting the middle bar can cause a boy to "see stars"); and
- not hanging out with others who want to hit the boy there.

Why do some kids want to hit me in my penis area?

Sometimes children think it is funny to hit others in their private area, but hitting someone in his/her private area is considered harassing behavior. If someone does this, the person being hit needs to tell the person to stop. If the person does not stop, the person being hit needs to talk with a trusted adult.

What is a sports cup for my penis?

A sports cup is an additional piece of sporting equipment that is worn by boys to protect their private area. Part of it is made of a hard material that covers a boy's penis and scrotum area under his clothing.

What is a jock strap?

A jock strap is made of specific materials to stretch around a boy's penis and scrotum. Its purpose is to keep a boy's private area in place, so it does not "jump around" while he is exercising.

Is it normal to have a crooked "dick"?

When erect, a boy's penis usually curves more to the right or left side. This curving does not mean his penis is crooked.

How big do penises get? Will my penis grow really BIG?

When not erect (not firm), a penis typically ranges in size from three and a half inches to five inches. When it is erect, or firm, a penis ranges in size from four inches to seven inches.

Does penis size matter?

No, penis size does not matter. The two main purposes of the penis are to release urine (pee) and carry sperm (found in the seminal fluids) out of a boy's body. So no matter what his penis size is, as long as the boy can release urine and seminal fluids, its size does not matter.

Do monkeys have penises?

Yes, male monkeys have penises.

Do cows have penises?

Male cattle, called bulls, have penises.

Do birds have penises?

Most types of male birds do not have penises. Instead, they have a lump called a cloaca to inseminate female birds.

Is There Something in Your Pocket or Are You Just Going Through Puberty? (Erections)

What is an erection?

An erection occurs when a boy's penis gets firmer (harder) and bigger because the capillaries, small blood vessels, in his penis fill up with blood.

Is there a bone in the penis? Is a "boner" a slang term for an erection that happens?

Some people use the slang term "boner" for an erect penis, yet there is no bone in a penis.

What year does your penis pop up?

Usually, a boy's penis can "pop up," become erect, anytime in his life. During puberty, erections occur more often when the boy is not expecting them, including as he sleeps.

If you get an erection, does that mean you're going through puberty?

A boy experiences more erections during his pubescent years, although his penis can get firm/hard at a younger age. The pleasurable feelings associated with erections are also understood more during puberty and the rest of the boy's life.

Am I weird because sometimes I wake up and my penis is hard?

Waking up with an erect penis is common for many boys. This occurrence does not mean boys are weird.

Can I pee if I wake up with an erection?

Most of the time a boy can still urinate upon waking up with an erect penis. To prevent hitting a wall or the floor with urine, he needs to hold/aim his penis more carefully towards the toilet.

Is it normal to have a boner of the penis when you have to take a wiz?

Sometimes a boy has an erection when he has to urinate. When this occurs, if he can urinate, he should carefully aim his penis to make sure urine goes into the toilet and not all over the floor and wall. If he cannot urinate, he needs to wait until his erection subsides.

Are you able to urinate when your excited penis is erect?

If a boy's penis is erect because he is thinking of something or someone pleasurable, he will be unable to urinate and needs to wait until his erection lessens.

After your penis grows (matures) and you think of someone you like, will it get bigger and harder?

Yes, a boy's penis may get longer and harder (firmer) when he thinks about someone he likes.

Why do we get erections when we are excited? Why do I get erections?

When a boy is excited, his heart beats faster and blood rushes into the blood vessels of his penis making it get firmer and bigger.

Why do we need to get an erection?

Erections are part of being a boy and experiencing them signifies he is growing up.

When do erections end (in a man's life)?

Males can usually continue to get erections for most of their lives.

Are there a certain number of erections to go through to be healthy for you? Are there a certain number of erections you get when going through puberty?

No, boys do not need to experience a particular number of erections during puberty. A boy can be healthy no matter how many erections he experiences.

How long does an erection last?

How long an erection lasts depends on the boy and the situation. If a boy is thinking of something or someone that made his penis erect and he wants the erection to go away, he can think of something else (something not exciting) to make his penis soft again. If he gets an erection and wants it to last (and he is in a private place), he can allow his penis to remain firm.

What do I do if my penis gets hard in class?

If a boy gets an erection during class, he can remain seated until it goes away. If he has to walk, he can carry a book or jacket/sweatshirt to cover the area.

How can I control my penis from getting hard?

Preventing erections depend upon the boy and the situation. If he is at a place where the erection is unwanted, like school, he can think of something to take his mind of off it, such as social studies homework, a math test, or a person like George Washington. As he gets used to the feeling of erections, the boy will learn how to prevent or control them at certain times. This awareness is part of growing up and becoming more mature.

Sailors and Their Little Swimmers (Semen and Sperm)

What is exactly cieman? *(Translation= What is semen?)*

Semen is the fluid that squirts out of the tip of the penis when a male ejaculates. It contains different fluids from the reproductive system, including sperm.

What are the fluids in ejaculate or "cum"?

Semen is made of fluids from the prostate and seminal glands, plus sperm.

What are some slang terms for semen?

Slang terms for semen include "cum," "love juice," and "sperm."

What color is semen?

Semen is usually a white or cream color.

What happens if I have purple cum?

Purple semen is uncommon. If a boy ejaculates purple semen, he should talk with a parent or other trusted adult to ask to speak to his doctor because he may have an infection.

My dad said he has green semen. Can semen be green?

Odds are your dad said his semen was cream colored (cream sounds similar to the word green). Yet if his semen is green colored, he should speak with his doctor.

What is sperm?

Sperm are cells released by a male when he ejaculates and are needed to fertilize eggs for creating babies.

Do sperm have tails?

Yes, the tails on the end of sperm help them to move.

Where does sperm form?

Sperm cells are created in the testicles, then stored in the epididymides (plural form of epididymis) located on the top of the testicles until needed.

Say if the sperm aren't needed?

Any cell a boy's body no longer needs is removed from his body through his excretory system.

Can a boy make sperm as a baby? Or as a little boy?

No, a boy cannot make sperm when he is a baby. Instead, his body begins to produce sperm when his body has grown to a certain point during puberty.

How old do you have to be to make sperm? At what age is the sperm made for us guys?

A boy's body is able to produce sperm when he reaches a certain level of physical maturity during puberty. The average age of this occurrence is eleven or twelve.

When do you stop making sperm?

Most men are able to produce sperm until an older age, although less sperm are found in each ejaculation.

Can I see sperm?

No, a boy is not able to see sperm in his semen with his bare eyes.

What are some signs of sperm?

A boy knows sperm came out of the tip of his penis when he ejaculates or has a wet dream.

How do I know that I am not peeing, but that it is sperm?

A boy can tell he has released semen and not urine by:

a. The fluid's color and smell: The fluid carrying sperm, semen, does not look or smell like urine. Semen is a white or cream color.
b. The amount of fluid: The amount of semen ejaculated is minimal in comparison to the typical amount of urine released when urinating.
c. The feelings he experiences: When semen is released, muscles in the private area contract creating a pleasurable feeling.

How long does sperm stay in the male's body if it isn't released?

Sperm are made and then stored in the epididymides for about two weeks.

Is it true that girls are born with eggs, but boys have to wait to produce sperm?

Yes and no. Girls are born with all their eggs, yet they are immature at birth. As they begin puberty, girls' eggs mature and are released until menopause. Regarding boys, they are born with some undeveloped cells, yet produce mature sperm for the first time during puberty. This mature sperm production can occur throughout a boy's life, in which sperm are continuously replenished (unlike girl's eggs).

"Did I Just Wet My Bed?" and Other Questions about Ejaculations

I woke up with wet pajamas and underwear. My bed was also wet. Did I just wet my bed?

Odds are a boy going through puberty who wakes up with damp underwear and pajamas did not urinate while he was sleeping. Instead, he probably had a wet dream.

What is a wet dream?

A wet dream occurs when a boy's semen, the fluid with sperm, comes out of the tip of his penis while he is sleeping. This occurrence is called a nocturnal emission meaning an emission that occurs while a boy is sleeping.

What is an ejaculation?

An ejaculation is the release of semen from a male.

Does a wet dream smell like pee?

No, semen has a different smell than urine.

Can I make myself have a wet dream?

No, a boy cannot go to bed and make himself have a wet dream. Instead, as he sleeps, his body decides to have an emission.

Are wet dreams bad? Are wet dreams harmful?

Wet dreams are natural occurrences for boys and are not bad.

Why do boys have wet dreams?

Boys have wet dreams as a way for their bodies to practice the release of semen.

How many wet dreams do boys have?

How many wet dreams a boy has depends on the boy. Some adult men remember having one or two wet dreams, others remember having more, and others do not remember having any when they were younger.

Can you be awake to have a wet dream?

No. If a boy is awake and releases semen, it is called an ejaculation.

Can a boy pee and ejaculate at the same time?

No, a boy cannot urinate and ejaculate at the same time. Once a boy has an erection because he is excited or turned on, the passageway from his bladder is blocked from releasing urine.

How much sperm comes out during an ejaculation?

The amount of sperm found in an ejaculation depends upon the boy's body and ranges from two hundred million to five hundred million sperm in each ejaculation.

Where is the sperm headed?

Where the sperm go depends upon what a boy is doing. If a boy ejaculates while he is sleeping (he has a wet dream) or masturbating, the sperm in his semen travels outside of his body onto whatever is around him. If a boy ejaculates while having sexual contact with a girl, the sperm try to find and fertilize an egg in the girl's body.

How long can sperm live?

How long sperm live depends upon where they are ejaculated. Sperm die within a period of time when released outside of the boy's body. If, though, semen (the fluid carrying sperm) is released into a female's body, sperm can live up to five days in her reproductive parts.

Other Curious Questions about Boys

How come my doctor asks me to cough when he touches my balls?

When going to a doctor's office for a physical, a boy may be given a hernia examination. To complete this exam, which takes only a few moments, the doctor holds the boy's testicles in his/her hand and asks him to cough as he/she feels for any movement in the boy's scrotum area. If a boy feels uncomfortable about this exam, he should talk with a parent or other trusted adult. He can also ask him/her to stay in the exam room with him as the exam is being performed.

What is a hernia?

A hernia occurs when the wall of an organ is weakened or becomes open in which the organ, or part of the organ, is no longer in its proper place.

My dad had a hernia. Will I get one?

Research shows hernias are hereditary which means if a boy's father had a hernia, the boy has a higher chance of also having one. Because of this increased chance, it is recommended boys have physical examinations on a regular basis.

How can a man get a hernia?
Sometimes a hernia happens naturally in the body. Other times they are caused when strain is put on the body.

How can I prevent a hernia?
To prevent a hernia, people can strengthen their core muscles (abdominal and back muscles) and be cautious when putting strain on their body. For example, people should always bend their knees when lifting heavy objects.

How do you get rid of a hernia?
An operation is usually needed to get rid of a hernia.

Can a boy live with a hernia?
A boy can live with a hernia, but it will be painful. Most men who have had a hernia recommend surgery.

Do boys have something like a period?
No, boys do not have periods because boys and girls have different reproductive parts.

Why does your penis hurt after you pee?
It is uncommon for a boy's penis to hurt after urinating. If this happens, the boy needs to talk with a parent or other trusted adult and then go to a doctor for a checkup.

What is masturbation?
Masturbation is the act of a person touching his/her private parts to feel pleasure.

Does sperm come out when you masturbate? Will that (ejaculation) happen when a boy plays with his penis?
When a boy masturbates, he may experience an ejaculation in which sperm is one part of this ejaculatory fluid.

Will a boy go blind if he touches his penis?

No. All boys touch their penis to urinate. And, if a boy touches his penis because it feels good to him, doing this will not make him blind.

I saw an advertisement for pills for old men. My dad told me they make a man get a hard penis. Why would a man take this?

The pills advertised on television are a prescribed medication some older men take to create erections because, as a man ages, he may have difficulty getting or keeping an erection.

Should boys our age use pills to make erections?

No, boys should not take any pill to create an erection because this medication is for older men who are in their fifties and older and under a doctor's care. Taking this medication when a boy is younger may damage his reproductive system and hormones.

What is a prostate?

The prostate is a gland located in a boy's reproductive system that releases fluid combining with other fluids to create semen.

What is prostate cancer?

Cancer can form anywhere in/on a person's body, in which some men have cancer cells form in their prostate gland. When this occurs, there are different procedures that can be done to remove the cancerous cells depending upon where they have appeared.

Is penis cancer real?

Yes, penis cancer is real.

Prepping Reminders

Both boys and girls are curious about the changes boys experience during puberty. Therefore, topics you can choose to prep for include:

- the changing of a boy's body shape,
- noticeable voice changes,
- new hair growth in facial, armpit, chest, and pubic areas,
- reproductive parts maturing, including penile growth, and
- nocturnal emissions (wet dreams).

Pregnancy and Babies

The following questions pertain to the curiosities children have about how babies are created and born. All are written in the manner asked by children, including the variety of ways the same type of question is asked. Within answers, the terms "female" and "male" are used instead of "girl" and "boy" to support the postponement of pregnancy by youth.

How a Baby is Made

How is a baby made? How do you have babies? How does the sperm get inside the woman?

A baby is made from two cells, an egg and a sperm. The egg is from a female and the sperm is from a male. The most common way for a female to get pregnant is for a male to ejaculate his semen, which has sperm, into a female's vagina. The sperm then travel through the cervix, the opening of the uterus, to find the egg to try to fertilize it.

Do babies form in your stomach?

No, a baby does not develop in a female's stomach. If this were true, the baby would be digested and then excreted, or removed, from her body. Instead, the baby forms in the female's uterus after one of her eggs is fertilized by a sperm.

How does a sperm know where to go? How do you get a sperm to the egg?

Just as certain parts of magnets are attracted to other parts of magnets, sperm are naturally attracted to eggs. Upon being placed into a female's vagina, sperm attempt to travel to find the egg by this natural "magnetic attraction."

Is the sperm finding the egg like an Easter egg contest?

In some ways a sperm finding an egg is like an Easter egg contest, yet there is usually only one egg for the sperm to find in the female.

How do sperm travel? How does a sperm travel up a girl's uterus?

Sperm travel by the movement of their tails.

How does the sperm get into an egg? How does an egg get fertilized?

Once sperm find the egg, they try to enter it by breaking into the egg's exterior.

How many sperm can fit into an egg?

Only one sperm can enter an egg.

How does an egg know to allow only one sperm in? Why can't two sperm or more enter an egg? Say if a sperm snuck in real fast after the first sperm entered the egg?

It is a scientific phenomenon—miracle—that the egg only allows one sperm inside itself. So, as soon as the first sperm enters the egg, the egg automatically closes itself up by hardening its outside so no other sperm can get in.

What does the rest of the sperm do after the egg is fertilized?

Remaining sperm are eventually excreted from the female's body.

How soon after people have sex do they get pregnant?

When pregnancy occurs depends on many factors, including where the egg has traveled to in the female's body and if sperm can travel to and penetrate into the egg.

My mom said I came from a lab. What does she mean?

A mom telling her child he/she came from a laboratory usually means some of her eggs were fertilized in a laboratory setting.

What is in vitro fertilization?

In vitro fertilization is a procedure done in a laboratory to combine an egg and sperm outside of a female's body. The basic steps include some eggs being removed from a female's ovary, fertilized in a sterilized container/dish, and then placed back into the female's uterus.

How many babies can a girl have?

How many babies a female can have depends on different factors. For example, if her body releases an egg regularly and a healthy sperm fertilizes it, a female can become pregnant each time this happens.

Can all women have babies? Can all men have babies?

Sometimes a female's or male's reproduction system does not allow the needed parts to create a baby. People who are in this situation usually discuss this occurrence with their doctors who can then provide additional information and options.

Experiences of Pregnant Females

How do most females first know they are pregnant?

Many females guess they are pregnant when their monthly period does not occur, yet this needs to be confirmed with a pregnancy test.

What is a pregnancy test?

A pregnancy test analyzes the urine (pee) of a female for a particular chemical. If this chemical is found in the urine, the female is pregnant.

How come the stomach gets bigger and the uterus does not?

It is the uterus, which is located in the middle of a female's lower abdominal area between her hipbones, that gets bigger as a baby grows inside his/her mother, not the stomach. And because there is limited room inside the mother's body, as the baby needs room to grow, the uterus begins to expand pushing towards the outside of the mother's body.

Why do pregnant women have to pee so much?

A pregnant woman urinates more often because the growing baby inside of her uterus pushes against her bladder.

My mom said that she got sick a lot when she was pregnant with me. Why is that?

It is thought that this happens because of the different chemical changes occurring in pregnant female bodies making some pregnant females feel sick in their stomach areas and, sometimes, causing them to throw up. This sickness is usually called morning sickness, although it can happen at any time of the day.

Why does what a mother eats affect the pregnancy?

What the female eats affects the pregnancy because whatever goes in her body travels to the uterus and baby.

Can a mom eat a lot of junk food when she is pregnant?

A pregnant female can eat some junk food, yet she needs to ensure she gets proper nutrition to help the growing baby in her uterus.

My aunt was pregnant and wanted to eat weird foods. Is that normal?

Yes, when some females are pregnant they crave certain foods that might be considered strange to others. As long as her body is okay with the food, she can eat it.

Should a mom smoke when she is pregnant?

Doctors recommend females to not smoke cigarettes or use other tobacco products while pregnant because the use of these products has been shown to cause possible health problems for babies.

Should a mom drink (alcohol) when she is pregnant?

Doctors recommend females to not drink alcohol while pregnant because the alcohol may negatively affect the pregnancy.

If you are pregnant, do you still have your period? Can you get your period when you are pregnant?

A pregnant female does not have her period until after the baby is born. She may, though, have some spotting in which some bloody fluid comes out of her vaginal opening. When this happens, she needs to check with her doctor to make sure she is okay.

Why do you have milk in your boobs after you have a baby?

After giving birth to a baby, the mother's brain releases a chemical telling her body the baby was born and needs nourishment (food). Milk then begins to form in her breasts to feed the baby.

Pregnancy and Youth

Can you have a baby at ten years old (at puberty)?

If a ten-year-old girl has started her menstrual cycle, she can get pregnant. This includes when she is about to release her first egg to have her first period.

Does going through puberty mean I'm ready to have a baby?

No, going through puberty allows a boy's and girl's body to grow to be able to have a baby. Yet this new ability does not mean he/she should have a baby.

I once read a story about a thirteen-year-old girl who is raising a baby. I would never do that. How bad is having a baby at that age?

There are some teenagers who have babies and raise them, making them responsible for another life, not just their own. Because having a baby at any age changes a person's life, many adults recommend teenagers wait until they are older and more mature for the responsibilities that come along with child raising.

I heard some young girl gave her baby to someone else to have. Why?

After giving birth, a female can give her baby to someone else to raise. This process is called putting a baby up for adoption. Deciding to do this is a difficult decision to make which is why it is usually recommended people wait to have a baby until they are mature enough to make life-changing decisions.

How a Baby is Born

How does a baby come out of a woman?
One way a baby is born is through a female's vaginal opening. Another way is through a C-section performed by a doctor.

How does the baby fit through your bottom?
A baby is pushed through the female's vaginal opening, not her buttocks/bottom. For this pushing, the female's vaginal opening stretches.

When you are getting ready to have a baby, does it hurt?
Yes, childbirth is usually painful. Many females who have given birth remember being in pain, but many believe the pain was worth it.

I was born by a C-section. What is this?
For a C-section, which means Cesarean section, a doctor makes an incision in the lower abdominal (belly) area of the mother, cutting through her skin, muscles, and uterus. The baby is then lifted out through the opening.

Is that why my mommy has a scar there?
Yes. If a female had a C-section, she has a scar in her lower abdominal area.

What is an afterbirth?
The afterbirth consists of the placenta and comes out of the mother after the baby is born.

Babies

How is it decided that a baby will be a boy or a girl growing in the mom?
The sperm cell determines if a baby will be a girl or a boy. Specifically, there is a part of the sperm with chromosomes that are "XX" for a girl or "XY" for a boy.

How do doctors know if a baby is going to be a girl or a boy?
When a female is pregnant, an ultrasound can be done in her lower abdominal area. By using this high-frequency sound wave machine, an

image of the growing baby inside her can be seen and, at a certain point during the pregnancy, the sex of the baby may be determined.

My grandmother said she can tell if a baby is going to be a boy or a girl because of how a pregnant woman looks. Is that true?

There are many myths existing about how to tell if a pregnant female is going to have a boy or a girl. The most accurate predictor is the sonogram. And the 100% correct answer is seen after the baby is born.

Why do movies show that the doctor wants the baby to cry after it is born? Is the doctor mean because he/she wants the baby to cry?

Having a newborn baby cry does not mean the doctor is mean. Crying allows the air passageway to cleanse itself and, when the baby cries, the doctor knows the baby is breathing on his/her own.

What happens when a baby doesn't cry when it is born?

If a baby does not cry or make other noises when he/she is first born, his/her airway passages need to be cleared with special equipment used by doctors and nurses.

Twins and Triplets

How are twins made?

There are two types of twins: fraternal and identical. Fraternal twins occur when two different sperm fertilize two different eggs. Identical twins occur when one fertilized egg (one egg fertilized by one sperm) splits into two parts.

If fraternal twins are born from one egg, how come their personalities, IQ, and ways they look are completely different?

The personalities, intelligent quotients (IQs), and looks of fraternal twins can be different because the two babies came from two different eggs and sperm (not one egg and one sperm).

How does the egg split in half for identical twins? When a woman is having identical twins, how does the egg divide?

For identical twins, the fertilized egg has the instinct to split itself in half in which certain chemicals in the cell help this separation to occur.

How are triplets made?

Most triplets occur when three eggs and three sperm combine (one sperm per egg). For identical triplets, which are less common, one egg splits into three parts.

My grandmother had twins. Does that mean I might have them too when I get older?

Anybody can have twins, yet the probability increases if certain blood relatives had them.

There are Many Types of Families

Is it important to give birth? Does everyone have to have a baby?

The choice to have a baby is personal in which some people choose to have a baby and others do not. Either choice is acceptable.

Can two men have a child? Can two women have a child?

Yes, two females can be parents and two males can be parents.

How can two women have a child together?

To get pregnant and give birth, one of the females needs to receive sperm from a man to fertilize the egg. This process can be done in a variety of ways. The females can also choose to adopt a child.

How can two men have a child together?

For two men to have a child together, they would adopt one.

Do people love adopted babies or children like their own?

Yes, people love their adopted babies and children as their own. Just because they did not give birth to a baby or child does not mean they will not love him/her as their own.

What are foster children?

Foster children are children who live with other people until their biological or adoptive parent(s) can take care of them again.

Are foster children adopted?

Sometimes biological and adoptive parents are unable to do take care of their children for an extended period of time, in which foster parents may then choose to legally adopt them.

Are foster children loved?

Yes, foster children are loved. Sometimes their biological or adoptive parents are unable to show love, yet children are often shown love by their foster parent(s) or other trusted adults.

Other Curious Questions about Pregnancy

Why do girls give birth and not boys? Can a male get pregnant?

Females can get pregnant and give birth because they have the reproductive system needed to have a baby and give birth. This system includes the vagina and uterus. Males do not have these parts and, therefore, cannot become pregnant, carry a baby, or give birth.

Why don't you have twenty babies at one time?

To have twenty babies at one time, females would need to release twenty eggs and have them fertilized or have one fertilized egg separate into twenty parts. This occurrence does not naturally happen in humans.

How does sperm touch the vagina if the penis goes through the girl's butt (in sex)? If someone is having intercourse through his or her backside and sperm goes in, will it get to the egg to fertilize it?

If any sperm are released by the entryway of a female's vagina, including the area by her anus, there is a chance for sperm to enter the vagina and travel to the egg.

Prepping Reminders

Children are curious about the process of having babies, just like we were when we were growing up. And, although some questions may cause you anxiety, by having a positive conversation with your child, he/she will see you as a trusted adult to return to for future questions and discussions.

Other Questions Commonly Asked During Puberty Talks

During discussions about puberty, teachers typically answer questions only about the topic. Yet it is common for children to ask other questions that deal with sexual activity or sexuality. Therefore, this section includes a variety of questions about these concepts and is written in the manner of how children may ask them.

If your child asks a question about sexual activity or sexuality, it is recommended you answer honestly and with age-appropriate terminology. By providing simple and honest answers, you are modeling truthful communication that is likely to encourage your child to approach you for future conversations.

Basic Questions about Sexual Activities

What is abstinence?
Abstinence means not engaging in a certain behavior. Regarding sex, abstinence means not having sex.

What is sex?
The word sex is used by some people to refer to a person's biological makeup of being a boy or a girl. Sex is also a term used to explain how a baby is made. When used in this manner, sex can refer to any act involving the genitals which includes the vaginal area for girls and the penile area for boys.

What is masturbation?

Masturbation is the act of a person touching his/her private parts for pleasure.

Can males or females masturbate?

Both males and females can masturbate.

Is it wrong to masturbate?

Choosing to masturbate is a personal choice and depends upon a person's values and comfort levels. Some religions or cultures discourage masturbation, yet others are okay with it.

Will masturbation hurt a person, like cause him/her to go blind or grow hair on his/her hands?

Masturbation does not typically cause harm to a person.

If a boy or girl touches him/herself during the school day, what should a teacher do?

If a boy or girl touches his/her private area in school, a teacher or other trusted adult needs to talk with the boy or girl to ensure he/she does not continue do this in school. Touching one's private area is private, which means if the boy or girl wants to touch his/her private parts, he/she should do this in a private (not public) place.

Why do people touch things (body parts) during kissing?

A person may touch body parts while kissing another person to give pleasure to himself/ herself or the other person.

What is a blow job?

A "blow job" is a slang phrase for fellatio, meaning someone uses his/her mouth on a male's penis to sexually stimulate or excite him. This behavior is a form of oral sex.

What is oral sex?

The phrase "oral sex" means a person's mouth is used on another person's genitals to excite him/her. Proper terms include fellatio, which means performing oral sex on a male, and cunnilingus, which means performing oral sex on a female.

What does it mean to "pop a girl's cherry"?

The phrase "pop a girl's cherry" refers to a girl having sexual intercourse for the first time. At this time, a girl's hymen may stretch, causing her to bleed.

Why do men have the urge to have sex?

Both men and women can have the urge to have sex because it is a natural instinct. Yet just because a person has an urge to have sex, it does not mean he/she should have sex.

Why is it unsafe to have sex?

Sexual activity can be risky because feelings about a partner can change unexpectedly causing emotional distress, a sexually transmitted disease may be passed, or an unexpected pregnancy may occur.

When is it safe to have sex?

Sexual activity is safer when both partners communicate honestly with one another, including having discussions about expectations, potential diseases, and taking precautions.

Is sex always bad?

If sexual activity were bad, there would not be so many people on the planet. Sexual activity can be pleasurable if people are mature with their partners, which includes talking honestly about sex and its consequences.

What is the main reason people even take the risk of having sex and possibly having a child?

People have sex because it is pleasurable and to have a baby. No matter what the reason is for having sex, people need to talk with their partner about possible consequences, both positive and negative.

How does it feel to have sex?

People say they experience a range of feelings when they have sex. Some may be pleasant, and others may be unpleasant due to a variety of reasons.

When you have sex for a long time, does it hurt?

Having sex for an extended period of time may hurt. If a person feels hurt or any pain, he/she should stop having sex and talk with a doctor.

What if your penis gets too big and it doesn't fit into a girl's private?

Most penises will fit into a female's vaginal opening because this area can stretch. If a female, though, is scared, does not want this to happen, or her vaginal area is not properly lubricated, the opening of the vagina can get tight making the entry difficult.

Can puberty give you of sexual super powers like in X-men?

No. Boys and girls will not get any sexual superpowers during puberty or any other time. They may have increased sexual thoughts, though, because the reproductive systems, which include the parts dealing with sex, are maturing. Also, hormones being released during puberty can make boys and girls more aware of these parts.

Legalities Pertaining to Behaviors, including Unwanted Behaviors

One of my friends told me he wanted to take a picture of my boobs. Is that alright?

No. Taking pictures of a young person's private parts is against the law. If a boy or girl is asked to have a picture taken, he/she should talk with a parent or other trusted adult.

My brother's girlfriend sent him a picture on his phone of her breasts. Will she get into trouble for that?

There are potential negative consequences for young people who choose to take pictures of their private parts and send them to others. Consequences include: having regret because other people have seen the pictures; no longer having a certain level of privacy; receiving penalties depending upon state law; and being denied entry into a college or business setting because the pictures were found online.

What is porn?

Porn is short for pornography. Examples of pornography include pictures and movies of naked people. In the United States, a person has to be eighteen years of age to watch or buy porn on television or the Internet.

Is it legal for a kid to have sex? Is there a legal age to have sex?

Each state in the United States has a law protecting young people from being victims of sexual crimes. This law notes the specific age a person has to be to give consent to sexual activity. If a boy or girl is under the specified age, he/she is considered a minor and not old enough to agree to have sex. And any person attempting to have sexual contact with a minor faces potential consequences, including legal trouble.

Would anything happen if my parent found out I had sex?

If a parent of a minor found out his/her son or daughter had sex, the parent can report it to police. And depending upon the age of the other person, he/she can have legal consequences.

Can children at sixteen (16) have sex physically? Like... are they able to do it?

Yes, most sixteen-year-olds are physically capable of having sex. Yet some people do not realize that having sex deals with feelings and responsibilities many sixteen-year-olds are not expecting. These include feelings changing after having sex in which the relationship may change, possible diseases, possible pregnancy, and what may happen if the other person tells others about having sex. Therefore, each person needs to think carefully about the decision to have sex.

Should children have sex?

Anybody choosing to have sexual contact with another person needs to consider all consequences. And because children are going through many challenges as they grow into adulthood, many people recommend young people wait to have sexual contact until they are older, which is why there are laws to protect minors.

What should I do if boys stare at my boobs during school?

Staring at a person's private parts, including breasts, is inappropriate. In school, staring at any person's private parts is considered sexual harassment. If this happens, the person who is being stared at needs to report the starring to a trusted adult, like a teacher, guidance counselor, nurse, or administrator.

If I don't want someone to touch me in my private area, what should I do if he/she tries to?

Attempt to say in a LOUD and FIRM voice "NO!!!" Then get away from the person as soon as you can, go to a safe place, and tell someone you trust. If you tell someone your age, ask that person to go with you to talk with a trusted adult for support and help.

I saw in a movie a man forcing a woman to have sex with him. Why would a man do that?

Most people are safe and do not cause harm to others. But some people may hurt a person, like forcing her or him to do something she or he does not want to do. If this happens, the victim, the person it happened to, needs to get help as soon as she or he can. Getting help includes telling a family member, the police, a doctor, or an emergency hotline about what happened.

Decision Making and Peer Pressure

What should I do about my friend peer pressuring me?

If a boy or girl feels pressure from a peer to do something unhealthy, he/she needs to talk with a parent or other trusted adult. The boy or girl can also talk with an older peer because someone who is older has usually experienced peer pressure and can give advice on what refusal skills to use.

My mom told me girls should be careful around boys. Why?

At times both boys and girls need to be careful around each other because sometimes one person suggests doing something unhealthy.

Why do girls pressure boys to go out with them?

Sometimes girls and boys see something in a movie or on a television show, or they get pressure from their peers about dating. Young people have to make the best decisions for themselves in which parents or other trusted adults can help a young person do that.

Why do boys pressure girls into having sex? Why do boys always want to make out and have sex?

Sometimes boys and girls hear or see something making them think they should be kissing and having sex. Sometimes they have feelings in their genitals, making them believe they want others to touch them there. But each person has to decide what is best for him/her. During puberty, there are many changes in a young person's life, including body development, more challenging schoolwork, and meeting new peers. Because there are many changes, it is recommended young people wait until they are older to have sexual contact.

But boys pressure girls to have sex. Why is that?

Sometimes a boy or girl may pressure another person to do something sexual because he/she is curious, has seen something in a movie or on television, or his/her friends have told him/her to have sex. But nobody should have sex unless he/she is sure having sex is the best decision for him/her. If a young person feels pressure to have sex, he/she should talk with a parent or other trusted adult. Also, each state in the United States has a law titled "age of consent" in which a person is unable to agree to engage in sexual activity until a certain age. The purpose of these laws is to protect young people.

What should I do if I feel pressured to have sex and I don't want to?

If you are pressured to have sex, you should look the person pressuring you straight in the eyes and say in a firm voice "No." If that person continues to pressure or make fun of you, immediately go to a safe place away from this person and talk with a parent or other trusted adult. "No" means "no."

Is it okay if I decide to wait until marriage to have sex? Do you think my friends will make fun of me?

Many young people decide to wait until marriage or a certain age to have sex because postponing sexual activity until a later age allows a person to mature. And regarding friends, real friends will not put down personal decisions but support them.

What happens if you like a girl/boy so much you want to have sex with her/him?

Liking someone does not mean a boy or girl should have sex. Yes, he/she might feel excited and attracted to the other person, but making the decision to have sex requires a person to be responsible and mature. This maturity includes answering the following questions in an honest manner before having sex:

- Why do you want to have sex?
- Are you of legal age to consent to have sex?
- How long do you expect to be in the relationship?
- How long does the other person expect to be in the relationship?
- Will you use protection to lower your chances of getting pregnant or getting an STD (sexually transmitted disease)?
- What will you do if you or the other person becomes pregnant?
- What will you do if you or the person gets a sexually transmitted disease (STD)?
- How will you feel if other people find out, including your friends or a parent?
- Are you emotionally ready to have sex?
- If you choose to have sex, how will you handle your emotions afterwards?
- Whom can you turn to if you need to talk with someone?

If a boy or girl is unable to seriously answer these questions or has different expectations than the other person, he/she should not have sex.

Terminology for Sexual Identity

What is biological sex?

Biological sex refers to the reproductive parts, chromosomes, and hormones a person has.

What is a chromosome?

Chromosomes help cells to grow and reproduce, making a person who he/she is.

Does a girl have different sex chromosomes than a boy?

Yes. A girl has two X chromosomes and a boy has one X and one Y chromosome.

What does intersex mean?

Intersex means a person was born with a combination of male and female biological aspects.

What is sexual orientation?

Sexual orientation is the phrase used to describe whom a person is attracted to.

What do heterosexual and homosexual mean?

Heterosexual is the term used for a person who is attracted to someone of the opposite sex. Homosexual is the term used for a person who is attracted to someone of the same sex.

What does it mean to be gay?

When a person is gay, he/she is sexually attracted to someone of the same sex. In other words, a boy is attracted to a boy and a girl is attracted to a girl.

How do you become gay?

People do not become gay, yet recognize they are gay. While growing up, youth become more aware of whom they are attracted to, noticing they may be attracted to someone of the same sex.

What does gender mean?

Gender typically refers to a person as being a male or a female in society.

A kid in my school is a boy but likes to dress like a girl. Is that okay?

Many schools support children dressing in a manner that expresses their gender. Some boys prefer to dress in what is considered more feminine clothing, and some girls prefer to dress in what is considered more masculine clothing.

What is gender expression?

Gender expression is the phrase used to describe how a person chooses to express who he/she is regarding masculinity and femininity.

What is gender identity?

Gender identity is the phrase used to describe how a person identifies him/herself as a man or woman.

Birth Control

What is a condom? What is a condom for?

A condom is a form of birth control that is placed over an erect penis to collect seminal fluid from an ejaculation. Using a condom lowers the risk of spreading sexually transmitted diseases and getting a female pregnant.

What is a condom made of?

Condoms are made from a variety of materials including latex, polyurethane, and lambskin. All of these products have the ability to stretch over an erect penis.

It is true that condoms can break?

Yes, condoms can rip or tear. To lessen the chances of this occurring, people need to follow the directions found on/in the condom packaging.

How old do you have to be to buy condoms?

There are no laws regarding age requirements for buying condoms.

Can we be shown in school how to use a condom?

Proper condom use is typically not demonstrated during puberty talks, but may be shown during sexuality discussions with teenagers if a school allows it. If a young person wants to learn how to use a condom, he/she can ask a parent or other trusted adult.

How do birth control pills stop the egg from being fertilized?

Depending upon their ingredients, birth control pills do one or both of the following:

- Stop the egg from being released from the female's ovary.
- Change the hormone levels in the female's uterus so an egg cannot be fertilized or attach itself to the wall of the uterus.

What is a vasectomy?

A vasectomy is a procedure done on a male to stop sperm from being released when he ejaculates. This procedure includes cutting or sealing the vas deferens from each testicle.

My mom has her tubes tied to not have babies anymore. What is that?

Tubal ligation is a procedure done in which the fallopian tubes of a female will no longer allow eggs to travel to her uterus.

Sexually Transmitted Diseases

What is an STD?

An STD stands for sexually transmitted disease, also known as sexually transmitted infection (STI) or venereal disease (VD). There are different types of STDs, which are caused by specific germs. They are called "sexually transmitted" because they are found in sexual fluids and can be passed through sexual contact.

Is an STD dangerous?

Some STDs are cured when a person takes medication. If medication is not taken, however, an STD can cause damage to a person's body. Examples of these STDs include chlamydia, trichomoniasis, and syphilis. Other STDs are incurable and remain in a person's body for his/her lifetime. Examples of incurable STDs are herpes and HIV (Human Immunodeficiency Virus).

Where do you go if you have an STD?

Anytime a person suspects he/she has an STD, he/she should go to a health clinic or doctor.

Can a sperm cause a disease in another person? If yes, how?

Semen, the fluid carrying sperm, can contain germs that cause sexually transmitted diseases (STDs). If a boy has a particular type of germ, like an STD, and another person has contact with his semen, he/she may also get the STD.

Can girls pass STDs to others?

If a girl has a particular type of STD germ and has sexual contact with another person, the other person may also get the STD.

My friend had a yeast infection. Is that an STD?

A yeast infection is caused by a fungus and can occur in the warm, moist parts of a person's body including the mouth, throat, vagina, and tip of the penis. Many yeast infections are caused by illnesses, stress, hormonal changes, and certain medications. Although yeast infections can be spread through sexual contact, they are not commonly caused this way and, therefore, not often thought of as an STD.

What is herpes?

Herpes is a virus that can create sores in the mouth and genital areas.

Can herpes get on a person's privates?

Yes, herpes is an STD that causes sores on a person's genitals. A person can get herpes by having sexual contact with someone else who has the herpes virus. Once the herpes virus enters his/her body, it remains there. In other words, there is no cure for herpes.

What is HPV?

HPV stands for the Human Papilloma Virus. This virus has many different forms (over a hundred) and can cause warts on some body parts and cancer in other body parts. The types of HPV dealing with the reproductive systems have been shown to cause genital warts and cancer of different reproductive system parts.

Can girls get HPV?

Yes, girls can get HPV. For girls, certain forms of HPV cause warts on the labia, rectal area, and inner thighs, as well as on internal reproductive parts. And some forms of HPV have been linked to cervical, vulvar, oral, and anal cancers.

Can boys get HPV?

Yes, boys can get HPV. For boys, certain forms of HPV cause warts on the penis, scrotum, rectal area, and inner thighs. And some forms of HPV have been linked to prostate, penile, testicular, oral, and anal cancers.

I have heard of girls getting a shot for HPV, and now there is a shot for boys. What does this shot do?

HPV vaccinations attempt to prevent a boy or girl from contracting the most common forms of the virus that cause genital warts and cancers of the reproductive systems.

Should I get this shot?

Getting any vaccination is a personal decision to talk about with a parent or other trusted adult. There are also resources available to help a person decide about vaccinations, including information from a doctor's office or reliable online resources.

What is HIV?

HIV stands for the Human Immunodeficiency Virus and is a sexually transmitted disease. Body fluids having high levels of this germ (virus) include the blood, breast milk, seminal fluids, vaginal fluids, and rectal mucous of people who are HIV positive.

How do you prevent HIV?

A person can prevent contracting HIV by not engaging in risky behaviors that can pass HIV. These risky behaviors include having sexual contact and/or sharing drug equipment with another person who is HIV positive.

Say if I know that I am going to have sex one day. Will I get HIV?

A person can only get HIV from another person who already has the virus. To prevent contracting HIV or any other STD, you and your potential partner should get tested for them at a clinic or doctor's office before having sexual contact. If the test results reveal someone has HIV or another STD, the clinician/doctor can provide additional advice.

Do condoms prevent HIV?

Condoms help to prevent HIV, yet they are not 100% effective. To ensure the highest effectiveness of a condom, users must carefully follow the directions provided in/on the condom packaging and use them consistently.

Can I get a disease from getting a tattoo or body piercing?

Diseases can be spread through improperly sterilized tattooing and body piercing equipment. Because of this risk, a person choosing to get a tattoo or body piercing should only go to a reputable establishment that has passed inspection by the local health department. In addition, only people trained in proper sterilization and disposal of equipment should be completing the work.

Seriousness about Sex

Why don't many people talk seriously about sex? Why are there so many jokes about sex?

The topic of sex makes some people feel uncomfortable and, therefore, they make jokes about it. That is why it is recommended for young people to talk to someone they trust and know will be honest with them when talking about sex.

If people can't talk seriously about sex, should they be having sex?

Sex needs to be taken seriously due to having positive and negative consequences. If someone cannot talk seriously about the topic and its potential consequences, this is typically a sign he/she is not mature enough to have any form of sexual contact.

Prepping Reminders

Children may ask questions found in this section during conversations about puberty. Although some questions may seem surprising, children are exposed to information, including sexual messages, within our society and are curious about what they see and hear. To be prepared (prepped), read over the provided questions and refer to other resources, like those provided in the back of this book. Also, consider talking with other parents about how to answer specific questions or about other concerns. By simply talking to another adult beforehand, your level of anxiety may lessen. And if you need to, reach out to a health professional for additional support.

Conclusion

I hope this book allowed you to have a better insight into what children are wondering about as they begin to go through the changes of puberty. I also hope the book gave you a better understanding of how questions can be answered in a simple, child-friendly manner. Although a parent's initial reaction may be to panic or feel distressed when his/her child grows older and shows curiosity, becoming a teenager is a natural part of your child's life. And, with guidance and support, children adjust to this stage of life in as healthy a manner as possible.

Points to remember:

- Children are naturally curious about life, including the body changes of puberty.
- Some children are anxious or scared about growing older. Having a trusted adult to listen to their fears and answer questions lowers their anxiety.
- Answering questions about puberty can be simple if the person answering takes his/her time and is honest.
- Although an adult may want to avoid talking about some aspects of puberty or sexuality, it is best for adults to be as honest as possible because children eventually learn the truth. And, upon learning an adult was not honest with him/her, the level of trust a child has towards that adult can be lowered.
- Along with puberty comes the personal decisions children make about life. For this, children need to hear the values of their family and community. Please share your values with your children.

Also, please note this book is one resource, in which it is recommended parents and other trusted adults seek additional support if needed. In other words, this book *does not* replace professional help. If needed, your child's doctor, school nurse, health teacher, or school counselor can help guide you to other specialists whose job is to provide support to parents and children. The job of a parent is vast which is why the proverb "it takes a village to raise a child" is true. Please ask for help when you need it.

I wish you and your child the very best... and a healthy puberty experience!

Resources

There are many resources available for parents and children on the topic of puberty and human sexuality. Some have reproductive system diagrams in either a paper or an online format. *Note:* Although using diagrams may feel awkward when talking with your child, having appropriate diagrams of body parts help children to learn about their bodies.

Books Written for Parents:

The Art of Talking with Your Teenager by Paul Swets (Adams Media Corporation, 1995).

Beyond the Big Talk: A Parent's Guide to Raising Sexually Healthy Teens - From Middle School To High School and Beyond by Debra Haffner and Alyssa Haffner Tartaglione (William Morrow Paperbacks, 2008).

Celebrating Girls: Nurturing and Empowering Our Daughters by Virginia Beane Rutter (Conari Press, 1996).

How to Talk So Children Will Listen & Listen So Children Will Talk by Adele Faber and Elaine Mazlish (Scribner, 2012).

How to Talk with Your Child about Sex: It's Better to Start Early, but It's Never Too Late by Linda Eyre and Richard Eyre (St. Martin's Griffin, 1999).

Sex and Sensibility: The Thinking Parent's Guide to Talking Sense about Sex by Deborah Roffman (Da Capo Press, 2001).

Ten Talks Parents Must Have With Their Children About Sex and Character by Pepper Schwartz and Dominic Cappello (Hyperion, 2000).

Talk with Me First: Everything You Need to Know to Become Your Kids' "Go-To" Person about Sex by Deborah Roffman (Da Capo Lifelong Books, 2012).

Books Written for Girls:

The Care & Keeping of You: The Body Book for Younger Girls by Valorie Schaefer and Josee Masse (Illustrator) (American Girl, 2012).

The Care & Keeping of You 2: The Body Book for Older Girls by Cara Natterson and Josee Masse (Illustrator) (American Girl, 2013).

Growing Up: It's A Girl Thing by Mavis Jukes (Knoft Books for Young Readers, 1998).

The Period Book, Updated Edition: Everything You Don't Want to Ask (But Need to Know) by Karen Gravelle and Debbie Palen (Illustrator) (Walker Childrens, 2006).

Ready, Set, Grow! A "What's Happening to My Body?" Book for Younger Girls by Lynda Madaras and Linda Davick (William Morrow Paperbacks, 2003).

"What's Happening to My Body?" Book for Girls by Lynda Madaras, Area Madaras, and Simon Sullivan (William Morrow Paperbacks, 2007).

Books Written for Boys:

Changes in You and Me: A Book About Puberty Mostly for Boys by Paulette Bourgeois, Kim Martyn, and Louise Phillips (Illustrator) (Key Porter Books, 2005).

My Body, My Self for Boys by Lynda Madaras and Area Madaras (William Morrow Paperbacks, 2007).

*On Your Mark, Get Set, And Grow!: A "What's Happening to my Body?"
Book for Boys* by Lynda Maderas and Paul Gilligan (William Morrow
Paperbacks, 2008).

***What's Going On Down There?** Answers to Questions Boys Find Hard to
Ask* by Karen Gravell, Nick Castro, Chava Castro, Robert Leighton, and
Walker & Co. (Walker Publishing Company, 1998).

"What's Happening to My Body?" Book for Boys by Lynda Madaras, Area
Madaras, and Simon Sullivan (William Morrow Paperbacks, 2007).

Books Written for both Boys and Girls:

It's Perfectly Normal: Changing Bodies, Growing Up, Sex, and Sexual Health
by Robie H. Harris and Michael Emberley (Illustrator) (Candlewick
Publishing, 2009).

It's So Amazing! A Book about Eggs, Sperm, Birth, Babies, and Families
by Robie H. Harris and Michael Emberley (Illustrator) (Candlewick
Publisher, 2014).

What's the Big Secret? Talking About Sex with Girls and Boys by Laurie
Krasny Brown and Marc Brown (Illustrator) (Little Brown Books for
Young Readers, 2000).

Where Did I Come From? by Peter Mayle and Arthur Robins (Illustrator)
(Lyle Stuart Inc., 2000).

Online Resources:

Advocates for Youth
Advocates for Youth focuses on the reproductive and sexual health of
young people and includes a Parents' Sex Education Center section. Found
at http://advocatesforyouth.org

BAM! Body and Mind
Created by the Centers for Disease Control and Prevention, this site is for children and focuses on a variety of health topics and decision-making skills. Found at http://www.cdc.gov/bam/body/body-smartz.html

Gay, Lesbian, & Straight Education Network (GLSEN)
GLSEN focuses on supporting respect for children in schools, no matter their gender identity, gender expression, or sexual orientation. Found at www.glsen.org

PBS Parents
The Public Broadcasting Service created this site for parents and includes information on child development. Found at http://www.pbs.org/parents/child-development/preteen-and-teen/

It's My Life
PBS Children created this child-friendly site focusing on a variety of age-appropriate topics, including puberty. Found at http://pbskids.org/itsmylife/body/puberty/

KidsHealth
Part of the Nemours Foundation's Center for Children's Health Media, this site has sections for parents, teens, and children on a variety of health topics. Found at http://www.kidshealth.org

The Scrub Club
Working with the National Sanitation Foundation International, this website has information regarding proper hand washing skills. Found at http://www.scrubclub.org/home.aspx

Stop It Now
This site provides programs and information on the prevention of child sexual abuse. Found at www.stopitnow.org

Online Resources with Child-Friendly Diagrams of the Reproductive Systems:

To find diagrams, type "reproductive system" in the web site's search engine.

Akron Children's Hospital at http://www.akronchildren.org

KidsHealth at http://www.kidshealth.org

Nationwide Children's Hospital at http://www.nationwidechildrens.org

About the Author

Once upon a time there was a health teacher named Lori A. Reichel who taught puberty lessons to preteens. For almost twenty years, this teacher was asked the same questions about what boys and girls should expect during their pubescent years. And, understanding children want and need to know what to expect, she provided her students with basic child-friendly, age-appropriate answers.

Throughout those years, Lori attended numerous workshops, trainings, and college courses, strengthening her skills in the classroom and as a health coordinator. These educational experiences led her to present at local, state, and national conferences, oversee wellness committees, and speak to administrators and educators about how to improve health education programs.

While presenting at her first state conference, another health teacher noticed Lori's teaching style and professionalism, and nominated her for a local award. A few months later, Lori received New York's Nassau County American Alliance for Health, Physical Education, Recreation, and Dance (AHPERD) 2004 Health Teacher of the Year Award. Then, in 2007, Lori received the New York State AHPERD Health Teacher of the Year Award. This was followed by the Eastern Division AHPERD Health Teacher of the Year Award in 2009, the National AHPERD Professional of the Year Award in Health Education in 2010, and the New York State AHPERD Professional of the Year Award in 2011.

In addition to helping children and other educators, Lori spoke with parent groups about how to talk with their children regarding puberty.

During these discussions, parents inquired what typical questions children ask on the topic. Many parents also expressed their anxiety about talking with their child on this topic, including feeling unsure of how to answer questions. Some asked for a resource, like a book, *just for parents* focusing on puberty.

Lori researched to find a particular resource for parents focusing only on the topic of puberty. What she found were books for parents written on the broad topic of sexuality and children's books on puberty. Recognizing the absence of a specific resource, this book was created specifically *for parents* with a focus on the *questions children ask about puberty*. Throughout the book, common questions children ask have been listed with child-friendly, age-appropriate answers. Also, questions children ask about pregnancy and basic sexuality are included because puberty talks may lead to questions on other sexuality topics.

In August 2013, Lori completed her doctorate degree in Health Education from Texas A&M University. Her dissertation topic focused on experiences parents face while talking with their children about sexuality topics, including puberty, as well as recommendations for what can be provided for parents. She currently is teaching at the University of Wisconsin-La Crosse in the Health Education and Health Promotion Department and continues to speak with parents regarding their experiences of teaching their children about sexuality topics.

If you are interested in contacting Lori, she can be emailed at pubertyprof@gmail.com and followed on Twitter at PubertyProf.

Index